CU00943342

Essential Stoma Care

Jennie Burch and Pat Black

St MARK'S
HOSPITAL

First published in the United Kingdom in 2017 by St Mark's Academic Institute, St Mark's Hospital, Northwick Park, Watford Road, Harrow, Middlesex HA1 3UJ.

Printed by Gwasg Gomer Cyf / Gomer Press Ltd, Parc Menter Llandysul, Llandysul, Ceredigion SA44 4JL.

Title: Essential Stoma Care

Authors: Jennie Burch and Pat Black

Copy-editor, designer and illustrator: Stephen Preston

ISBN: 978-0-9935363-1-1

Contents

Introduction

This book was written by two nurses who have a combined total of over 60 years working in colorectal nursing, with much of that time being stoma specialist nurses. This book is written for healthcare professionals and to provide an overview of stomas.

In this book the chapters are designed to address details about stomas; each chapter ends with a reference list that can be used for further reading on the topic if required. The book takes the reader from the basics such as what a stoma is, to why they are formed and includes a discussion on the role of the stoma specialist nurse. Each of the three main output stomas are then addressed in turn, enabling the reader to understand the reasons for the formation of each stoma type, what operations may be undertaken and the appropriate appliances needed. Any special considerations for a person with a stoma are also explored to include colostomy irrigation, diet for a person with an ileostomy and support groups. The final chapter explores complications that can occur with a stoma or the skin around it, stoma reversal and also quality of life.

Patients who are to have a stoma formation or who already have a stoma often travel a difficult path; understanding this will enable healthcare professionals to provide better care for this group of patients. The book has been reviewed by Professor Sue Clark who is a colorectal consultant surgeon at St Mark's Hospital.

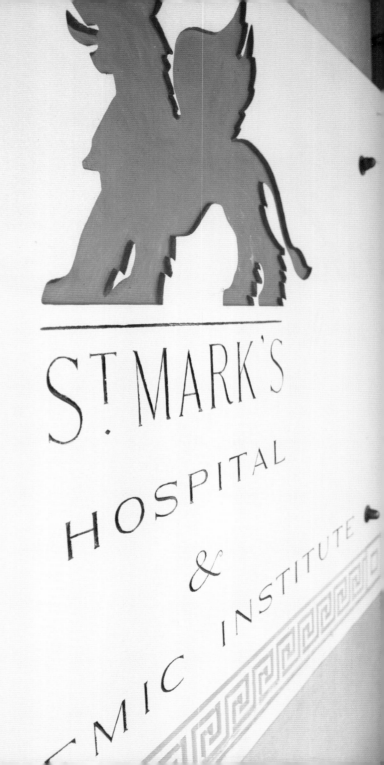

St. MARK'S

HOSPITAL

&

EMIC INSTITUTE

Chapter 1: Background

History of stomas

The evolution of the stoma can be traced far back through history with the pre-Christian Israelites being aware of the problem of abdominal injuries and the consequences of the spillage of 'dirt'. In the Bible (Judges 3, v.21–23) Eglon, the King of Moab, is stabbed by Ehud (see *Fig. 1.1*).

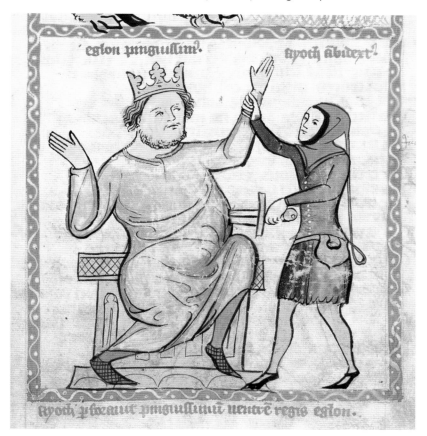

Fig. 1.1: King of Moab being stabbed by Ehud: 'He took the dagger and thrust it into his belly and the shaft went in after the blade so that he could not draw the dagger out of his belly and the dirt came out'.

Celsus (55BC–AD7) quoted by Dinnick (1934) noted that if the small bowel had been penetrated nothing could be done. However, he felt that if the large bowel could be sutured then all would not be lost. Output of the artificial anus or stoma was considered by Lord Chesterfield to be defined as 'dirt' and as such, was matter out of place (Black 2000).

From the middle of the nineteenth century until the present day, the basic concept of colostomy construction has remained unchanged, although many technical improvements have taken place. One improvement by Hartmann in 1923 was the elective resection of the rectosigmoid cancer with formation of a left iliac fossa colostomy. Miles followed in the 1920s with the abdominoperineal resection.

What is a stoma?

Stoma comes from the classical Greek word meaning mouth or chasm and in medical terms, artificial opening. A stoma is a surgically formed opening where the bowel is exteriorised through the abdominal wall to enable the faecal output to be eliminated from the body. There are three main types of output stoma: the colostomy, ileostomy and urostomy. There are other types of stoma such as the tracheostomy and jejunostomy. A tracheostomy can be described as a surgical opening in the anterior wall of the trachea to help with ventilation often in conjunction with a tracheostomy tube. A jejunostomy can be an opening out of the jejunum where the bowel is formed into an output stoma, but this is rare and will require nutritional supplementation due to the physical lack of bowel. A jejunostomy can also be a method of feeding: a plastic jejunostomy tube is placed through the skin of the abdomen and into the small bowel at the level of the jejunum to deliver food and medicine if the person cannot eat by mouth.

The colostomy, ileostomy and urostomy are explained and explored in their own separate chapters. This will include why they are formed, how they are formed, the usual output from the stoma and other issues related to each type of stoma. The people with a stoma can be termed ostomates or ostomists or more specifically colostomate, ileostomate and urostomate.

There are several generic terms that are associated with a stoma. These are loop, end and double-barrelled.

Loop stoma

The loop stoma can appear larger and bulkier than an end stoma as it has two openings.

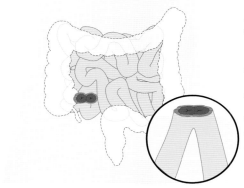

A loop of bowel is brought through the abdominal wall and formed into a stoma, which can be round or egg shaped.

The proximal loop will pass faeces and the distal loop will pass mucus (see *Fig. 1.2*). This tends to be a temporary stoma.

Fig. 1.2: loop stoma

End stoma

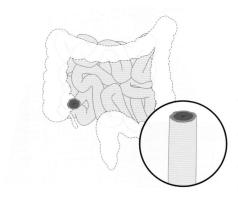

An end stoma is a segment of bowel that is bought through the abdominal wall and formed into a stoma which tends to be round in shape.

The other end may be removed or left inside the body, depending on the operation.

This can be a permanent or temporary stoma (see *Fig. 1.3*).

Fig. 1.3: end stoma

Double-barrelled stoma

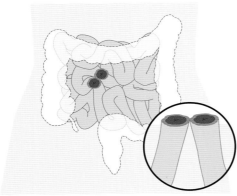

When forming a double-barrelled stoma, the surgeon divides the bowel completely (see *Fig. 1.4*).

Each opening is brought to the surface as a separate stoma; one is the distal end and the other the proximal end.

The two stomas may or may not be separated by skin.

Fig. 1.4: double-barrelled stoma

Stoma statistics

It is estimated that there are approximately 120,000 people in the UK with a stoma, which equates to about 1 in 500 people (Boyles and Hunt 2016). The NHS website states that about 6,400 new permanent colostomies are formed each year in the UK and about 9,000 new ileostomies are formed yearly. The vast majority of people in the UK with a stoma have a colostomy but there are an increasing number of people with a temporary ileostomy due to the advances in anal sphincter saving operations.

Anatomy and physiology

The skin is the largest organ in the body, with multiple layers. The outer layer of the skin is the epidermis, below this the dermis and hypodermis.

The skin has a number of functions including defence from the entry of bacteria; this requires the skin surface to be intact.

There are a number of appendages associated with the skin including sebaceous glands, sweat glands and hair, all of which can prove problematic to the person with a stoma in relation to the adherence of stoma appliances if excessive. Shaving or trimming the hair can assist with appliance adhesion.

The abdomen

The abdominal wall has the outer layer of skin, which covers the superficial fascia that is formed from fibrous connective tissue and superficial fat and below this are the abdominal muscles. There are a number of these muscles: the internal and external obliques, the transverse abdominis and the rectus abdominis. These muscles perform a number of tasks: they protect the organs inside the abdomen and can increase the intra-abdominal pressure that is necessary for defecation, for example.

It is common practice to site the stoma through the rectus muscle as it is thought to reduce the risk of a parastomal hernia. Lining the walls of the abdominal cavity is the peritoneum, which is a large serous membrane. The mesentery carries blood vessels, nerves and lymphatics to the organs and attaches many of the intra-abdominal organs to the abdominal wall.

The gastrointestinal tract

The gastrointestinal (GI) tract, also termed the alimentary canal, is a complicated organ that begins at the mouth and ends at the anus (see *Fig. 1.5*). It is basically a muscular tube that is about nine metres in length.

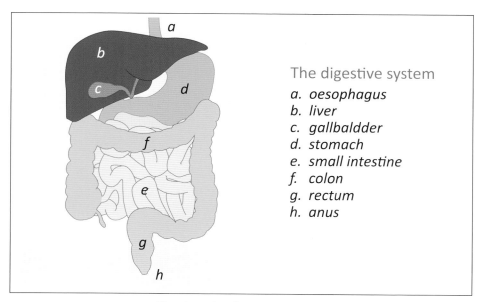

The digestive system

a. *oesophagus*
b. *liver*
c. *gallbaldder*
d. *stomach*
e. *small intestine*
f. *colon*
g. *rectum*
h. *anus*

Fig. 1.5: the digestive system

The function of the gastrointestinal tract

The function of the GI tract is to ingest, digest and absorb food and then eliminate waste (Black and Hyde 2005). This process includes secretion by the accessory organs such as the salivary glands and the gallbladder of about seven litres of fluid per day into the GI tract to breakdown the food by chemical means. The food is propelled along the GI tract involuntarily by ripples in the muscles of the bowel wall termed peristalsis; backflow is prevented by several sphincters, such as the ileocaecal valve. This is the mechanical digestive process to help break apart and mix the food into a bolus; peristalsis ceases for a period of time following surgery. The bowel mucosa secretes mucus, hormones and digestive enzymes.

Once the food has been broken down, the nutrients are absorbed from the bowel lumen, via the mucosa, into the lymph or blood supply. There is little absorbed in the stomach except alcohol. Most absorption occurs in the small bowel; this includes litres of fluids as well as nutrients such as proteins broken down into amino acids. In the last section of the ileum vitamin B12 is absorbed and if this part of the bowel is resected during surgery the person may require supplementation of vitamin B12. In the colon further fluid is reabsorbed and also sodium.

The waste in the form of the faeces is eliminated from the body through the anus or stoma. Part of this waste is the epithelial cells of the stomach and intestine that are rapidly renewed every week or so.

The small bowel

The first section of the bowel (also termed intestine) is the small bowel, which is the majority of the length of the GI tract and consists of the duodenum, jejunum and ileum. The main function of the small bowel is to absorb nutrients. This is enabled by the villi and folds within the mucosa that increase the surface area and thus the potential to absorb nutrients, including amino acids, fatty acids and saccharides. The secretions from the liver, gallbladder and pancreas are necessary for the breakdown of food.

When absorption occurs from inside the small bowel, glucose and sodium are drawn across the epithelium with the fluid. This is important when considering rehydration therapy for people with a high output stoma, which requires glucose to absorb the sodium. If there is an extensive small bowel resection, it might mean that it is not possible to absorb adequate nutrition from the diet to sustain life. Additionally there can be damage to the villi with starvation, radiotherapy or coeliac disease, potentially producing a high faecal output and a reduction in the absorption potential.

The large bowel

The large bowel consists of the caecum, ascending, transverse, descending and sigmoid colon; also the rectum and anal canal (see *Fig. 1.6*). The colon is about 150 cm in length and the primary function is the absorption of water and electrolytes until the waste becomes formed faeces. Although most of the water is absorbed in the small bowel, about 1000 ml is absorbed by the colon until the faeces are reduced to about 150 g daily.

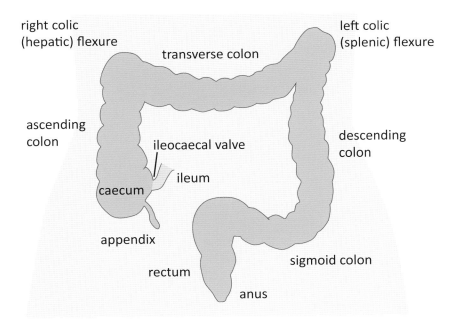

Fig. 1.6: the large intestine

The caecum joins the ileum at the ileocaecal valve; the valve prevents backflow of the waste from the colon back into the ileum. Also in the caecum is the appendix. As faeces travel along the ascending colon the faeces thicken as water is absorbed, along with sodium, potassium, chloride and glucose. The corner of the bowel where the ascending colon meets the transverse colon is the hepatic flexure, which lies next to the liver. In the transverse colon mucus from goblet cells in the epithelium lubricates and protects the bowel. The transverse colon passes around the splenic flexure to the descending colon, near the spleen. The descending colon leads to the sigmoid colon and finally the rectum.

When faeces reach the rectum a signal is sent to indicate that faeces can be passed; whether this occurs or not is under the control of the person. At this stage the faeces are usually solid and can be several days from when food was ingested. The longer the faeces are in the colon the drier they will be. To pass faeces it must travel via the anal canal. Faecal continence is controlled by two anal sphincters. Faeces are made of indigestible matter that has been ingested and also dead bacteria and cells shed from the bowel lining.

Within the bowel there are bacteria, some of which are important within the digestive process and will produce vitamin K for example. There is risk of infection during bowel surgery as the bacteria can leave the bowel and enter the abdominal cavity. The bowel flora changes as a result of antibiotics and this may result in an infection such as clostridium difficile. The bacteria also ferment carbohydrate and produce methane gas, as much as 500 ml each day (Richards 2005). A high fibre diet can increase flatus production. Flatus also can be malodorous and potentially a problem for people with a colostomy.

The gastrointestinal blood supply

The blood supply to the GI tract includes the mesenteric arteries. The superior mesenteric artery (SMA) supplies oxygenated blood to the jejunum and ileum and the blood supply needs to be carefully preserved during surgery.

Rarely an infarct of the SMA occurs which can result in a necrotic bowel which often requires an extensive small bowel resection. The venous blood supply contains nutrients that pass through the hepatic portal vein, a possible route for metastatic bowel cancer spread.

The urinary system

The urinary system consists of two kidneys, two ureters, a bladder and the urethra. There are three main functions of the urinary system which are excretion, elimination and homeostasis.

The kidneys

The two kidneys are either side of the spine with the right one slightly lower than the left (see *Fig. 1.7*).

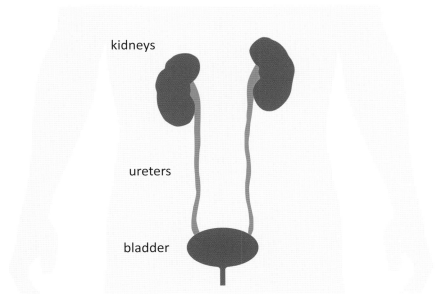

Fig. 1.7: the kidneys

The kidneys receive 1000 ml of blood each minute (Mirpuri and Patel 2000). The function of the kidneys is to maintain homeostasis by regulating body fluids, sodium and blood pressure levels. The kidneys also produce urine, getting rid of metabolic waste from the blood and they secrete hormones. Urine is produced in a number of stages; the blood is filtered and the majority is reabsorbed. The amount of reabsorption is controlled by anti-diuretic hormone (ADH) that is secreted by the pituitary gland. Within each kidney are over a million tiny tubules that are termed nephrons which filter the blood and transfer the filtered fluids.

The ureters

There are two ureters, one from each kidney. The ureters are 30 cm long muscular tubes that are only about 3 mm in diameter. The function of the ureter is to transport urine from the kidney to the bladder by a series of peristaltic contractions occurring several times each minute.

The bladder

The bladder is a reservoir to contain urine with the ureters entering at the base of the bladder; backflow of urine is prevented by muscles at the ureteric openings. The bladder fills with urine until there is about 200–400 ml; at this stage the desire to urinate is felt. The bladder can hold over 500 ml but discomfort will usually be felt.

The urethra

The urethra is the passage from the bladder to the external urethral opening. In females the urethra is about 4 cm long whereas in men the urethra is about 20 cm long. In men the urethra is also used as part of the reproductive system. Urinary continence is maintained by sphincters.

Urine

The normal amount of urine passed each day is 1–2 litres and urine is ideally amber coloured fluid. The volume and colour of urine can vary depending upon fluids consumed and sweating for example. The specific gravity of urine should be 1015 to 1025 and the pH about 7.4. Urine consists predominately of water, with some salts, urea and creatinine.

Diseases that may result in the formation of a stoma

There are numerous diseases or conditions that might result in the formation of a stoma; the more common are colorectal cancer, bladder cancer, diverticular disease and inflammatory bowel disease.

Colorectal cancer

The third most common cancer in the UK is colorectal cancer. There are about 40,000 people in the UK diagnosed with colorectal cancer each year (Patnick and Atkin 2011). Older people are more likely to have colorectal cancer than younger people and more people are surviving after treatment. The symptoms of colorectal cancer include rectal bleeding, a change in bowel habit and weight loss, although these symptoms may be associated with many less serious problems. The cause of colorectal cancer is not fully understood but smoking, alcohol consumption and a diet high in red meat and processed foods are thought to increase the incidence. It is also thought that eating high levels of fruit and vegetables and physical activity may be protective against colorectal cancer.

Most colorectal cancers develop from a benign adenomatous polyp within the bowel and change over a period of many years into a cancer. Thus there is the potential to remove the polyp before it becomes cancerous. If a colorectal cancer spreads it is likely to metastasise to the lymph nodes and liver and possibly other sites within the body. Cancers are generally staged using the TNM classification, where T=tumour, N=nodes and M=distant metastasis. Prior to this classification the Dukes' staging was used; A, B and C with several subcategories added later. If a patient has a T1N0M0 staging this means that the tumour is confined within the bowel and has not spread to the lymph nodes or anywhere else in the body. There is more than a 90% survival rate five years after treatment for people with this grading (Whyte et al 2011).

Some people require surgery to treat their bowel cancer which may or may not result in the formation of a stoma. In addition to surgery some people require chemotherapy or radiotherapy. If treatment is prior to the operation it is termed neoadjuvant therapy; after surgery it is called adjuvant therapy. Often it is unnecessary for people to undergo preoperative therapy if the resection margins are clear or not threatened. This means that the cancer has not spread to areas that cannot be removed during the operation. In this situation surgery is often advocated first. If, after the operation, the tumour is categorised as a T1 or T2 without positive margins (all the cancer was removed and there was no cancer left at the edges) and there were no positive lymph nodes, chemotherapy is not recommended after the operation.

Bladder cancer

A bladder cancer can be described as a growth of abnormal tissues in the bladder lining. A cancer of the bladder is less common than a bowel cancer and can often be locally excised; if the bladder requires removal it will result in the formation of a urinary diversion. This will be discussed in Chapter 4.

Government statistics suggest that there are about 10,000 people diagnosed with bladder cancer each year, making it the seventh most common cancer in the UK. The causes of bladder cancer are linked with smoking and exposure to certain industrial chemicals. It is more common in older adults and men are more commonly affected than women. The staging of the cancer is similar to the bowel cancer staging and is TNM, where T is tumour, N is related to nodal involvement and M is related to the spread of cancer to other body organs such as the bones, lungs or liver.

Diverticular disease

Diverticular disease is common, affecting the majority of elderly people. Diverticular disease is the presence of small pockets that protrude from the colon, most commonly the sigmoid colon, which weakens the bowel wall. About half of people over the age of 50 have these small pockets (diverticula) and they cause symptoms such as abdominal pain if they become inflamed. The causes of diverticular disease are linked with low fibre diets and constipation. In rare cases these small pockets can burst, allowing the contents of the bowel to leak into the abdominal cavity causing peritonitis which will require emergency surgery, usually a Hartmann's procedure (discussed in Chapter 2).

Inflammatory bowel disease (IBD)

Inflammatory bowel disease is an umbrella term for Crohn's disease and ulcerative colitis, two distinctly different but linked bowel diseases. The former affects any part of the gastrointestinal tract from the mouth to the anus, while ulcerative colitis only affects the rectum and colon. The symptoms include abdominal pain and diarrhoea. The causes include genetic and environmental factors. The majority of people are treated with drugs but surgery may be necessary, most commonly removal of the affected area of bowel such as the colon.

Necrotising enterocolitis

Necrotising enterocolitis (NEC) is predominately seen in the pre-term neonate and has a mortality rate of 30–50%. NEC is acute necrosis of the gut involving the area of the distal terminal ileum. On rare occasions the whole of the ileum and colon may be affected. NEC occurs because the bowel has become injured through an ischaemic event such as birth asphyxia or congenital heart disease. Most often an ileostomy is fashioned for NEC in the neonatal period and occasionally in older children for small bowel obstruction, perforation or necrosis associated with intra-peritoneal sepsis. The use of loop stomas may be contraindicated as they tend to have a higher incidence of complications, do not fully defunction the distal bowel and applying a stoma bag can be more difficult.

Hirschsprung's disease

Hirschsprung's disease occurs in approximately 1 in 5,000 births and causes intestinal obstruction. The absence of ganglionic cells in the distal large bowel causes lack of innervation to that particular part of the bowel. In 80% of neonates with Hirschsprung's disease the problem is located in the rectum and sigmoid colon.

Sometimes the problem is not noticed until several days after birth and if the disease is present in a mild form, diagnosis can be delayed until the child is older. In approximately 25% of neonates, Hirschsprung's disease presents with intestinal obstruction, abdominal distension and vomiting (Black 2000).

Colostomies formed for Hirschsprung's are usually placed in the proximal sigmoid or descending colon and within ganglionic bowel confirmed by frozen section biopsy at the time of surgery and as close as possible to the distal aganglionic segment. Sometimes with neonatal operations, stomas can be placed within the laparotomy wound. It has been shown that this method has an acceptably low incidence of complications and has the advantage of requiring only one incision at the time of closure. Stomas brought out separately from the wound are just as effective although slightly more difficult to secure and have an increased incidence of stoma stenosis, but a slightly lower incidence of wound sepsis.

Imperforate anus

One of the common anorectal malformations seen is imperforate anus. Anorectal malformations occur in approximately 1 in 5,000 births and are slightly more common in males. These malformations can occur with other defects and can be classified as low, intermediate or high defects. Imperforate anus is usually identified immediately after birth by the midwife during routine examination.

Immediate surgical intervention is needed to create a bowel diversion, usually a loop colostomy and then further radiological tests are undertaken to discern the extent of the lesion. After correction of a low or high lesion the stoma is reversed and a new anal opening created. The parent is taught how to do dilatations of the new anal canal regularly to ensure patency.

Stoma guidelines

The ASCN UK (Association of Stoma Care Nurses) is currently writing guidelines about a variety of different topics to guide the care of people with a stoma. These can be accessed at the website **ascnuk.com** which requires a small yearly membership fee. There are two main documents that are available from this newly formed group: the nursing standards and audit tool and also the ASCN clinical guidelines. The latter document offers information on colostomy irrigation and discharge guidelines among other topics.

There are also guidelines on caring for some of the more common stoma-related complications that occur, such as managing high output stomas and preventing formation of a parastomal hernia.

Although these documents offer some guidance it is not possible to determine the care for all people with a stoma in a totally prescriptive manner as the needs can vary dramatically depending on the individual.

Role of the stoma specialist nurse

The role of the nurse who cares for people with a stoma can be a stand-alone role or can incorporate other roles such as colorectal cancer. The ASCN (2015) defines the role of the stoma specialist nurse to include:

- Preoperative preparation for potential/actual stoma formation
- Postoperative stoma care management, including practical and psychological care
- Preparation for discharge from hospital
- Support at home

Preoperative care

In elective surgery, it is ideal for patients to be seen and counselled in preparation for their operation. The nurse explains about the stoma, what it looks like, how it will act and how to care for it. The nurse will also discuss many other topics, such as the care plan whilst in hospital. It is also recommended to start training patients on their stoma care before surgery

(Chaudhri et al 2005). With ERAS (enhanced recovery after surgery) pathways, many patients are only in hospital for a few days after their operation, so using the 'fake' stoma in the preoperative training pack has been shown to be effective in allowing safe discharge home after five days (Bryan and Dukes 2010).

Stoma siting

The stoma specialist nurse will also mark the site where the surgeon will form the stoma during the operation (see *Fig. 1.8*). This requires a process of assessments of the abdomen, the rectus muscle and any changes in the abdominal shape when moving positions.

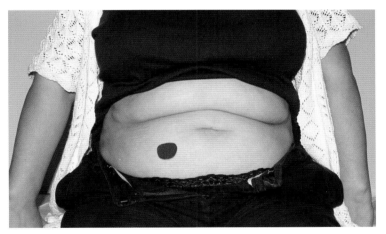

Fig. 1.8: marked stoma site

There are a variety of principles related to stoma siting that need to be adhered to such as avoiding creases in the abdominal wall and ensuring that the patient can see and reach the stoma site (Burch 2008).

Postoperative stoma education

In the postoperative period patients need to be reminded of preoperative information given to them, such as about diet and exercise. One of roles of the nurse in the postoperative period is to ensure that the person with a newly formed stoma is able to care for their stoma independently.

The appliance should be carefully removed from the abdomen without damaging the skin. The skin around the stoma (peristomal skin) needs to be gently but thoroughly cleaned, most often with warm tap water and carefully dried. Finally the new appliance needs to be applied to the skin around the stoma, with the hole in the appliance (the aperture) being cut to the appropriate size.

The aperture needs to be made a few millimetres larger but to the same shape as the stoma. The appliance should be carefully applied so that the adhesive is around the stoma and the stoma is within the aperture. The appliance should be held in position for 30 seconds with the hand to help it to adhere well to the peristomal skin.

The patient also needs to be educated to recognise changes in the peristomal skin; the skin should look the same as the rest of the abdominal wall, free from redness or skin breaks. If this changes patients should contact their nurse for assessment and treatment if needed.

Kristensen et al (2013) consider that learning how to change the stoma appliance is the beginning of independence and acceptance of the stoma. However, despite this there is no method that is formally recognised to assess when the patient has become proficient in the self-management of their stoma.

Thus they determined a seven point evaluation scale to monitor how well the patient was coping in these domains:

- How the patient reacts to the stoma
- Removing the appliance
- Measuring the stoma size
- Adjusting the size as required
- Skin care
- Fitting the new appliance
- Emptying the appliance

The nurse rates the patient out of four for self-care for each of these stoma skills. They acknowledge this is only the start of learning to live with a stoma but consider the newly devised instrument can act as a good tool for assessing when patients become able to self-manage their stoma.

In emergency situations patients are often more unwell than in elective cases and may also have peritonitis, for example. Additionally they will usually miss out on the important stage of preparation for surgery. It is thought that many patients who undergo emergency surgery initially do not cope so well physically and emotionally with their stoma and often need greater levels of help and support after surgery.

Discharge planning

It is important to plan a safe discharge home for all surgical patients. Plans need to include generic factors such as whether the patient is medically well enough to be discharged, so blood results and observations should be satisfactory. In relation to stoma care it is important to ensure patients have adequate and appropriate stoma stock levels, are independent with their stoma care and have contact numbers for stoma help once at home.

Additionally it is important to know what to do should a problem occur and what is and is not allowed in the initial postoperative period once at home. This can include avoiding heavy lifting, but walking is encouraged to improve general fitness and well-being.

Advice such as about bathing and swimming is also important. Patients can take a bath or shower with or without a pouching system in place. Normal exposure to air and water will not harm the stoma. Water will not flow into the stoma. Soap will not irritate it, but soap may interfere with the skin barrier sticking to the peristomal skin. People with a stoma can swim in a swimming pool, sea or lake. They do need to make sure that the appliance is empty and secure before swimming. After swimming and drying some patients choose to apply a new appliance. Swimming in a public place without an appliance in situ is not allowed.

Stoma care follow-up

There is uncertainty regarding how, what and when stoma care follow-up should be arranged. Follow-up can be a telephone call, a home visit or a nurse-led clinic appointment. It has been suggested that a telephone call within the first week of being discharged home is ideal (Davenport 2014). Although patients have a contact number it is thought that many do not call or do not recognise that they need to call for advice and guidance. In many areas home visits are undertaken, but with restriction on budgets this is not always possible. A home visit does enable the nurse to undertake a full assessment, including assessing how well the patient is coping once they are back in their home environment and how they are adapting to life with a stoma.

A clinic visit can enable a full assessment of the patient and if there are any complications the nurse will often have treatments that they can use to improve the situation. Clinic appointments can also be organised to coincide with the surgical or medical appointment to save multiple trips to the hospital. Due to the high number of possible complications associated with a stoma life-long follow-up is required. Furthermore, as stoma appliances are expensive, the nurse needs to ensure that they are appropriately used. Mangall et al (2013) describe the cost of stoma appliances accounting for over 2% of the clinical commissioning group prescribing budget.

Care of the elderly person with a stoma

The elderly person can struggle to maintain an acceptable standard of existence due to comorbidities and diminishing faculties (see *Box 1.1*). Illness and surgery, particularly stoma surgery can make their lives more challenging.

Box 1.1 - Issues that may affect coping with a stoma

- Hearing
- Sight
- Speech
- Confusion
- Memory loss
- Hemiplegia
- Paraplegia
- Arthritis
- Parkinson's disease
- Obesity
- Pendulous breasts
- Aging skin
- Loss of body fat

Some elderly people may have had a stoma many years ago and grown old, but now are having difficulty with the appliance, or may have moved into a care home where the staff are unsure how to care for the individual. Some older people may live in their own home or a residential home and become ill suddenly and find they need surgery and a stoma. There may be difficulties in counselling the older patient due to hearing problems or a missing hearing aid. Many have memories of relatives or friends who had surgery in earlier years, when having a stoma was surrounded by stigma. They may remember the smell because at that time the stoma appliances available did not adhere as well as modern appliances and sometimes people had to make do with gauze or cotton wool over the stoma. Also when the older patient is seen preoperatively they may worry about talking to a young nurse, who may seem no older than their grandchildren, about their bowels, which they may see as an intrusion to their privacy.

Postoperative problems

After surgery there may be confusion due to anaesthetics and analgesia. Teaching often has to be at a slower pace and will frequently have to be repeated (see *Box 1.2*). An easy to use appliance is helpful and it is important to use an uncomplicated routine and remember that the patient's intellectual function may be slow.

Box 1.2 – Ways to help an elderly person become proficient with their stoma care

- Multi-sensory teaching
- Allow recovery time
- Motivate by independence
- Ensure privacy and quietness
- Choose best time for teaching
- Set realistic goals
- Gain attention
- Have extra aids available - glasses, mirror and instruction card
- Allow time to comprehend information

The elderly person may have a poor sense of smell which may prevent the patient from detecting an appliance leakage.

Some patients who are still ill after surgery and who are not coping with their stoma care may not be able to return to their own home and discussion should be started about how best to care for them. Many may have families who are keen to look after the patient to help them recuperate but the patient may not be keen on the idea as it may be a long way from where they live. Some want to be in their own home to be able to sort out their personal matters and put their affairs in order.

If there is a chance of a step down facility before going home this is useful as it will help the patient to have more time in a less rushed atmosphere to enable them to take control of their stoma care routine as soon as possible.

It is always important to try and involve the family, after discussion with the patient, regarding whether they want their partner or other family member to help with the stoma care. It should never be assumed that the partner or family member will automatically assume the role of carer. There may be the need for a discussion about some help for the patient, sometimes needing someone to either cut the flange or help with flange placement, especially if the patient has sight problems or dexterity issues.

Dehydration can be a big problem as the elderly may fear urinary incontinence if they drink too much. Lack of fluid may lead to a urinary tract infection making the problem of looking after the stoma more difficult. Antibiotics may cause diarrhoea and there may be the need to use a drainable appliance while the medication is being taken. Also for the elderly person with an ileostomy, particularly if they have a poor renal function, dehydration can cause problems that may result in readmission to hospital.

Cooking and eating when living alone can be a problem. Often individuals cannot be bothered and exist on sandwiches because it is easier. Shopping may be difficult as well. Meals on wheels could be recommended and depending on money, Wiltshire Foods service is a useful standby.

Unfortunately false teeth are often misplaced in hospital and this causes a problem with eating, only allowing the patient to have a soft food diet, which may cause the stoma to be more active and potentially leak.

Other problems

The individual may have dementia or Parkinson's disease, which may render the patient unable to undertake their own stoma care or understand what to do. There may be problems during or just after surgery and the patient may have had a cerebral vascular accident (CVA) and be unable to care for their stoma. Patients who had a stoma some years before may suffer disease recurrence and need further surgery. Sometimes only palliative surgery can be offered, simply to form a stoma to divert faeces away from an obstructing bowel tumour.

Paediatric stoma care

A stoma in a neonate can be extremely distressing for the parents especially if it is needed for a congenital malformation. The stoma in the neonate is often temporary whereas the stoma in the older child may be permanent. Today, invasive abdominal surgery in children under five years old is not carried out in local district hospitals, but in specialised children's units. It is estimated that eighty per cent of childrens' stomas are raised shortly after birth with one in ten in the first year of life and the remaining ten per cent before the age of eighteen years.

Stoma site

The site of the stoma formation is determined by the patient's specific diagnosis. For individuals with long-term or permanent stomas, the site of the stoma becomes an essential feature of the surgery performed. A poorly sited stoma can be difficult to manage as the child grows. The stoma specialist nurse in conjunction with the surgeon should choose and mark the most suitable site prior to the operation. In the neonatal period this is more difficult because of abdominal distension and the frequent urgency of surgery.

Skin care and appliances

Neonatal skin is very fragile and great care needs to be taken with the application and removal of stoma appliances. There is a greater ratio of surface area to body weight and chemicals in skin care products can be absorbed through the skin. The peristomal skin can be easily traumatised but as the infant's gestational age increases, the pre-term infant's skin becomes more similar to adult skin. The use of products containing benzyl alcohol, especially for neonates in incubators, should be avoided. In 1982 it was discovered that there was a link between products containing benzyl alcohol and cardiovascular collapse of neonates in incubators, subsequently named as 'the gasping baby syndrome'. Consequently, the Food and Drugs Agency and the American Academy of Paediatrics recommended that benzyl alcohol-containing products should be avoided in infant usage (Lesney 2001).

One-piece appliances are usually the most suitable (in a paediatric size) and they are lightweight. A pre-term infant or young baby will find a two-piece appliance heavy and even a lightweight paediatric appliance on a very tiny pre-term infant (less than 2 kg) can be heavy enough to cause difficulty with the infant's breathing, taking into account all the other tubes that may also be on the skin.

Often the easiest way of caring for a faecal stoma in a tiny pre-term infant is to use petroleum jelly around the peristomal area and cover the stoma with a very light piece of gauze with a layer of petroleum jelly on the gauze also. Frequent changes of the dressing should be done. The stoma specialist nurse will often teach the parents how to care for their infant in the special care baby unit.

Often once surgery is done and the infant is stable, they are returned to their local hospital baby unit and the stoma specialist nurse will liaise with the community paediatric team for stoma care and support of the parents. One of the common worries for nurses and parents is the stoma changing colour to either blueish or even white. This happens when the infant pulls up their knees and contracts the abdominal muscles when crying and the contracted muscle momentarily traps the bowel.

As the infant grows and starts to walk, a two-piece appliance may be more useful and easier for the parents to manage. As the child reaches school age there may need to be a discussion with the school and nursery carers about the care of the stoma while the child is at school. If the school is unfamiliar with a child with a stoma the stoma specialist nurse may the best person to work with the parents and the school to help all parties understand the needs of the child.

Manufacturers

Within the UK there are many stoma appliance manufacturers. Some of these are summarised in *Table 1.1* with their websites. Some of these companies also delivery stoma products to the patients' homes each month when they receive the prescription for the stoma equipment.

Company name	Website
B. Braun Medical UK	bbraun.co.uk
Bullen Healthcare	bullens.com
CliniMed	clinimed.co.uk
Coloplast UK	coloplast.co.uk
ConvaTec	convatec.co.uk
Dansac Ltd	dansac.co.uk
Eakin	eakin.eu
Hollister Limited	hollister.co.uk
Oakmed Ltd	oakmed.co.uk
Pelican Healthcare	pelicanhealthcare.co.uk
Respond	respond.co.uk
Salts Healthcare Ltd	salts.co.uk
Trio Healthcare	triohealthcare.co.uk

Table 1.1 stoma appliance manufacturers

References

Association of Stoma Care Nurses UK (2015) Stoma care nursing standards and audit tool. ASCN UK. London.

Black PK (2000) Holistic stoma care. Baillière Tindall. London.

Black PK and Hyde CH (2005) Diverticular disease. Whurr Publishers. London.

Boyles A and Hunt S (2016) Care and management of a stoma: maintaining peristomal skin health. British Journal of Nursing. 25(17): S14–S21.

Bryan S and Dukes S (2010) The enhanced recovery programme for stoma patients: an audit. British Journal of Nursing. 19(13):831–834.

Burch J (2008) Stoma care. Wiley-Blackwell. West Sussex.

Chaudhri S, Brown L, Hassan I and Horgan AF (2005) Preoperative intensive, community-based vs traditional stoma education: a randomized, controlled trial. Diseases of the Colon & Rectum. 48(3):504–509.

Davenport R (2014) A proven pathway for stoma care: the value of stoma care. British Journal of Nursing. 23(22): 1174–1180.

Dinnick T (1934) The origins and evolution of colostomy. British Journal of Surgery. 22(85): 142–154.

Kristensen SA, Laustsen S, Kiesbye B and Jensen BT (2013) The urostomy education scale: a reliable and valid tool to evaluate urostomy self-care skills among cystectomy patients. Journal of Wound Ostomy and Continence Nursing. 40(6): 611–617.

Lesney S (2001) More than just sugar in the pill. Today's Chemist. 10(1): 30–6.

Mangall J, Lakin S, Burke D and Midgley K (2013) An alternative model of prescribing stoma appliances. British Journal of Community Nursing. 18(10): 485–91.

Mirpuri N and Patel P (2000) Renal and urinary systems. Mosby. London.

Patnick J and Atkin WS (2011) Screening for colorectal cancer. In: Young A, Hobbs R and Kerr D (eds) ABC of colorectal cancer. 2nd edition. Wiley-Blackwell. West Sussex.

Richards A (2005) Intestinal physiology and its implications for patients with bowel stomas. In: Breckman B (ed) Stoma care and rehabilitation. Elsevier Churchill Livingstone. London.

Whyte S, Chilcott J, Cooper K, Essat M, Stevens J et al (2011) Re-appraisal of the options for colorectal cancer screening. University of Sheffield, School of Health and Related Research (ScHARR) Sheffield.

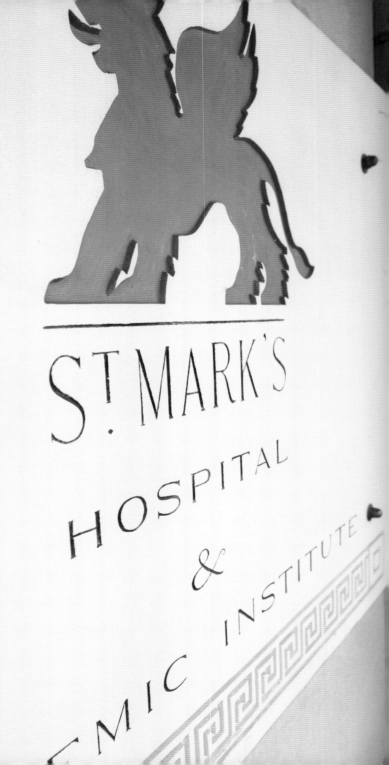

Chapter 2: Colostomy

What is a colostomy?

A colostomy (see *Fig. 2.1*) is formed from the colon. The bowel is stitched onto the abdominal wall and the skin around the stoma heals in the normal way. The stoma is the bowel and visually it is red, slightly wet and shiny. This is how a healthy stoma should appear; similar to the mucosa (lining) on the inside of the mouth.

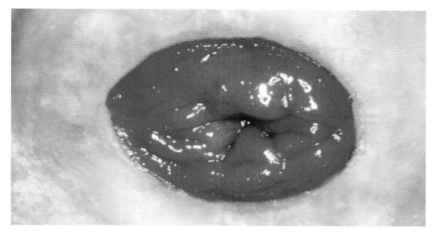

Fig. 2.1: a colostomy

The normal colostomy output is soft, formed faeces. A colostomy is usually active between three times a day and three times a week. Flatus will also be passed. The output is collected in a closed appliance that is replaced when about a third full (Burch 2008).

A bowel movement through a colostomy is like a normal movement through the anus but it cannot be controlled as it would be if it was going through the anus. Unlike the anal opening, the colostomy does not have sphincter muscles that can stop or hold the passage of stool. This means there must be an appliance over the stoma to collect anything that might come through, whether it is expected or not.

There are many lightweight appliances that do not show under clothes. Stoma appliances stick to the skin around the colostomy and are generally worn all the time.

Some people with a descending or sigmoid colostomy find that by eating certain foods at certain times, they can make the bowel move at a time that works best for them.

Some people use only this method to keep bowel movements on a regular schedule, while others may use it along with colostomy irrigation. A transverse colostomy will usually put out stool at all times no matter what is eaten and when it is eaten. The firmness of the stool is affected by what is eaten and drunk.

Why is a colostomy formed?

There are many reasons for colostomy formation. Some of these can be seen in *Box 2.1* (Black 2000).

Box 2.1 – Conditions that may require a colostomy formation

- Colorectal cancer
- Diverticular disease
- Crohn's disease
- Radiation proctopathy
- Ischaemic colitis
- Faecal incontinence
- Trauma
- Congenital conditions, e.g. Hirschsprung's disease

What operations result in a colostomy formation?

Colostomy construction is often more difficult than ileostomy construction. Patients who have a colostomy formation, particularly for colorectal cancer, may be older and fatter which creates a bulky colon. To ensure adequate length of colon it may be necessary to mobilise the splenic flexure and left colon (Norton et al 2008).

Abdominoperineal excision of the rectum

Abdominoperineal excision of the rectum (APER, APR, AP, eLAP) can be performed for cancer of the rectum or anal canal where the cancer is close to or infiltrating the anal sphincter. This procedure involves an abdominal wound(s) and a perineal wound with a permanent colostomy (see *Fig. 2.2*). The lower sigmoid colon, rectum, anal canal and sphincter muscles are all removed. In some cases this may be done via laparoscopy. Complications that may arise are poor perineal wound healing, urinary dysfunction and sexual dysfunction, although these are less of an issue with modern surgical techniques.

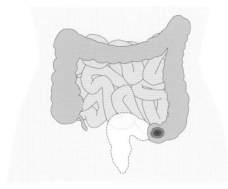
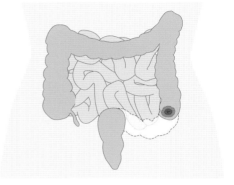

Fig. 2.2: permanent colostomy   *Fig. 2.3: Hartmann's procedure*

Hartmann's procedure

A Hartmann's procedure is basically the removal of the sigmoid colon (see *Fig. 2.3*). This procedure is usually performed in the emergency situation when it is unsafe to re-join the bowel ends (anastomose), thus a temporary end colostomy is performed. This is often reversed at a later stage when and if the patient is better.

Transverse colostomy

The transverse colostomy (see *Fig. 2.4*) is formed in the upper abdomen, either in the middle or toward the right side of the body. If there are problems in the lower bowel, such as an obstruction, the patient may be too ill at that stage to have a full resection therefore a transverse colostomy may be formed to keep stool away from the colon that is inflamed, infected, obstructed, or newly operated on to allow healing to take place. This type of colostomy is usually temporary.

A permanent transverse colostomy is made when the lower portion of the colon must be removed or permanently rested, or if other health problems make the patient unable to have more surgery. The colostomy is then the permanent exit site for stool and will not be closed in the future.

The faeces that comes out of a transverse colostomy varies from person to person and even from time to time.

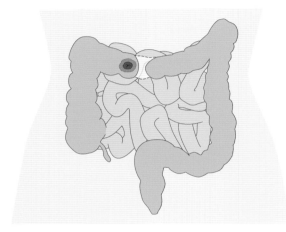

A few transverse colostomies put out firm stool at infrequent intervals, but most of them move fairly often and put out soft or loose stool.

The faeces contain digestive enzymes much like an ileostomy output and can be corrosive to the skin near the stoma.

Fig. 2.4: transverse colostomy

Colostomy appliances

Colostomy appliances are available in one and two pieces (see *Fig. 2.5*), in transparent or opaque material.

A two-piece appliance has a separate flange and bag enabling the flange to be left on the skin for between one and three days while the bag can be changed as often as necessary (Lee 2001). This keeps the peristomal skin intact and risk of the skin stripping is reduced.

One-piece appliances have a flange that is attached to the bag (integral) and flange and bag are removed together in one action. Colostomy bags will have a filter at the top of the appliance that allows flatus to slowly disperse to stop the appliance 'ballooning'. Stoma bags have a skin-friendly adhesive ring (flange) and are soft against the skin due to the covering of the appliance. Colostomy bags can be worn in the bath or shower as they dry very easily when exiting. If using a one-piece appliance it may need to be changed more than once a day as there is no drainable end on a colostomy appliance.

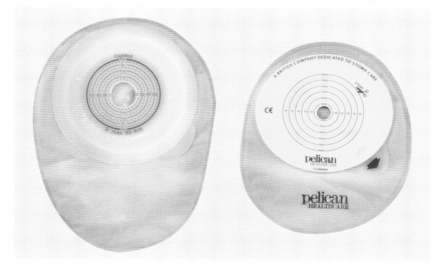

Fig. 2.5: colostomy appliances

Colostomy irrigation

Colostomy irrigation is suitable for people with a descending or sigmoid colostomy (Osbourne et al 2013). Irrigation allows the introduction of water into the colon through the colostomy to empty faeces and flatus via the colostomy and to help to regulate bowel movements. Whether to irrigate depends upon a number of factors including the patient's wishes after a full discussion with the stoma specialist nurse.

Whether a patient irrigates their colostomy and how to do it depends on many factors, such as:

- The amount of bowel that is left in situ
- Patient motivation
- Patient skill and comfort level with irrigation
- Suitable facilities will be needed at home i.e. toilet facilities, privacy, bathroom facilities
- What neoadjuvant or adjuvant therapy the patient may have had

It will take time to set up a routine. Daily irrigation is usually required to ensure that there is no 'breakthrough' of faeces between irrigations.

Equipment needed

The stoma specialist nurse will teach the patient how to irrigate the colostomy with the specialist irrigation equipment (see *Fig. 2.6*) that is available on prescription:

- A plastic irrigating container with a long tube and a cone
- An irrigation sleeve to carry the irrigation output and faeces into the toilet
- A sleeve closure clip and a belt for extra irrigation sleeve support

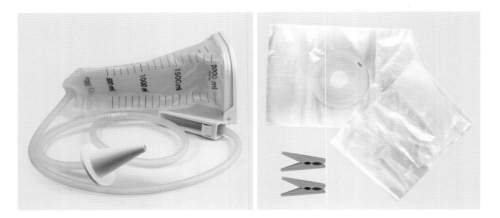

Fig. 2.6: specialist irrigation equipment

When to irrigate

The patient should choose a time in the day when the bathroom will be free for a period of time. Irrigation may work better if it is performed after a meal or a hot drink and irrigation should be done at the same time of day to obtain regularity.

How to irrigate

Patients should be advised to:

- Prepare all the equipment beforehand
- Clamp the tubing and put 1000–1500 ml of warm (not hot) water in the irrigating container. NEVER connect the tube directly to the tap
- Hang the container above shoulder height
- Sit up straight on the toilet or on a chair next to it
- Seal the plastic irrigation sleeve over the colostomy and put the bottom end of the sleeve in the toilet bowl
- Remove air bubbles from the tubing by opening the clamp on the tubing and letting a small amount of water run into the sleeve
- Wet the end of the cone or lubricate it with water-soluble lubricant
- Put the cone into the colostomy as far as it will go comfortably
- Slowly open the clamp on the tubing and allow the water to flow into the colostomy. It takes several minutes to drip in 300–500 ml of water
- Check continually that the water is going into the colostomy and NOT into the toilet
- The amount of water needed will depend on each patient and in time they will understand how much they need. Less may be needed, but do not use more than 1000 ml. The purpose of irrigating is to remove stool, not to be strict about the amount of water used
- Hold the cone in place for about ten seconds after all the water has gone in
- After the water has run in, remove the cone. The faeces will come out in spurts over the next 30–45 minutes
- As soon as most of the stool has come out, fasten the bottom of the irrigating sleeve to the top with a closure clip. The patient is then free to move around, bathe or do anything else to pass the time
- It can be advisable to have a hot drink in this period
- With time and experience the patient will get to know when all the water and stool have come out. A squirt of gas may be a sign that the process is done or the stoma may look quiet or inactive
- When all the faeces and irrigation fluid has left the colostomy apply the stoma cap/plug
- Rinse irrigation equipment; the bag, cone and sleeve and hang to dry

Problem solving

- Cramps or nausea should not be experienced while the water flows in. These are signs that either the water is running in too fast, that too much water is being used or that the water is too cold. After the water has been put into the colostomy, a bowel movement-type cramp may occur as the stool comes out
- If the complete irrigation process always takes much more than an hour the patient should be reviewed and assessed by the stoma specialist nurse to see why
- There are potential concerns that softened water will have a high salt content and can be dangerous when used to irrigate. There will always be one mains water tap in the house that is not connected to the water softener
- While learning how to irrigate, it is often advisable for patients to wear a stoma appliance rather than a cap or plug until they are confident that the colostomy is inactive

Stoma plug

For a colostomy patient to be able to use a stoma plug it is important that the stoma output is formed and that there are no more than two bowel actions per day, as the plug's action is to hold back faecal waste until the bowel can be evacuated. The plug, which is mushroom-shaped, is inserted into the colostomy and the patient is taught to increase the time each day that the plug is used, starting off with an hour at a time. As the time frame increases, the plug can be used for up to twelve hours a day. After the plug has been removed and evacuation has taken place, a new plug or a colostomy appliance may be used.

Diet for a person with a colostomy

Everything that is eaten or drunk serves as fuel for the body. To stay in good health, the body needs carbohydrates, proteins, fats, minerals and vitamins. Water is also a key part of good health. At least 8–10 glasses (about 250 ml) of water a day is usually recommended with a normal diet. Having a balanced diet helps maintain good nutrition and keep the bowels activity normal.

There is no such thing as a diet for people with a colostomy. After healing is complete and the colostomy is working normally, most people with a colostomy can return to their usual diet which should be chewed well. Those foods that have disagreed with a person prior to colostomy forming surgery may still do so.

It is advisable to try a food that seems to disagree with patients three times. If after the third time the food still seems to have an adverse effect the patient will often choose to avoid it in their diet. Patients on a special diet because of heart disease, diabetes or other health problems should ask their doctor or dietitian (a referral is required) about a diet that will be suitable.

Patients soon learn which foods produce gas or odours (such as cabbage), which foods cause diarrhoea (such as spicy food) and which lead to constipation (such as low fibre foods). It is possible to regulate the bowels behaviour to some extent; however it is not possible to prevent the bowel from moving by not eating.

An empty bowel still produces gas and mucus. It is therefore advisable for patients to eat regularly, several times a day and this will encourage the colostomy to function well. That said, people with IBS (irritable bowel syndrome) symptoms such as alternating constipation and diarrhoea prior to the colostomy formation are likely to persist after the colostomy is formed.

Pharmacological considerations with a colostomy

For some colostomy patients, prescribed and over the counter drugs may have unwanted side-effects on the gut and affect the output of the stoma. There are many different drugs that can affect colostomy function:

- Drugs that affect the function of the gut via the autonomic nervous system are cholinergic drugs and adrenergic drugs such as atropine, belladonna, dicyclomine hydrochloride, hyoscine and propantheline bromide
- Drugs that have a direct action on the gut are analgesics (such as codeine phosphate), antibiotics, laxatives, antacids and ion-exchange resin
- Drugs that have an indirect action on the gut are sedatives, diuretics and digoxin
- Drugs which may cause gut disturbance are the tricyclic antidepressants such as amitriptyline, doxepin, nortriptyline, protriptyline and trimipramine

- Some commonly used or prescribed hay fever preparations or antihistamines can affect the gut with anti-cholinergic affects such as cyclizine, promethazine and diphenhydramine
- Monoamine oxidase inhibitors may cause constipation
- Laxatives come in many varieties and their main effect is to increase stool frequency. There are a variety of different types of laxatives:
    - Solid bulk laxatives are agar, bran, isphagula, methylcellulose and sterculia
    - Osmotic laxatives are lactulose, magnesium salts and sodium salts
    - Lubricant laxatives are liquid paraffin and dioctyl sodium sulfosuccinate
    - Stimulant laxatives are senna, cascara and bisacodyl

Occasionally the patient or nurse may see whole tablets discharged into the stoma appliance and this will often worry the nurse or patient. Some of the drugs are formulated with a wax matrix and the impregnated drug in the wax matrix is leached out during the passage of the drug through the gut. The most common modified release tablets are Burinex K, Centyl K, Esidrex K and Navidrex K.

Specific care needs for a person with a colostomy

There are a number of specific needs for a person with a colostomy in relation to the bowel output. This is usually soft and formed but can be constipated or diarrhoea.

Diarrhoea

It is possible to have an upset stomach when on holiday or at home so it is advisable for a person with a colostomy to have a small supply of drainable appliances. These can then be drained as needed instead of being taken off each time the bowel is active, which can be excessive if unwell. This can help to prevent sore skin occurring around the stoma, as a result of frequently removing the appliance, which can also be called skin stripping as the top surface of the skin is removed.

Constipation

If a person was prone to constipation prior to the colostomy being formed it is likely that this will continue after the operation. It is easier to prevent constipation than treat it when a colostomy is present, as although it is possible to use treatments like a suppository or enema, these do not stay inside the colostomy very well and may not be effective. Nurses can advise patients to have a balanced diet including adequate amounts of fibre, fluids and exercise. If this is not enough laxatives can be tried.

Support groups

The main national support group in the UK for people with a colostomy is the colostomy association.

They have an informative website **www.colostomyassociation.org.uk**. There are many local support groups also available.

References

Black PK (2000) Holistic stoma care. Baillière Tindall. London.

Burch J (2008) Stoma care. Wiley-Blackwell. West Sussex.

Lee J (2001) Nurse prescribing in practice: patient choice in stoma care. British Journal of Community Nursing. 6(1): 33–37.

Norton C, Taylor C and Nunwa A (2008) Oxford handbook of gastrointestinal nursing. Oxford University Press. Oxford.

Osbourne W, Bowles T, Hanley J, Tomsett G and Williams J (2013) Stoma care nursing standards and audit tool. ASCN UK (Association of stoma care nurses UK). London.

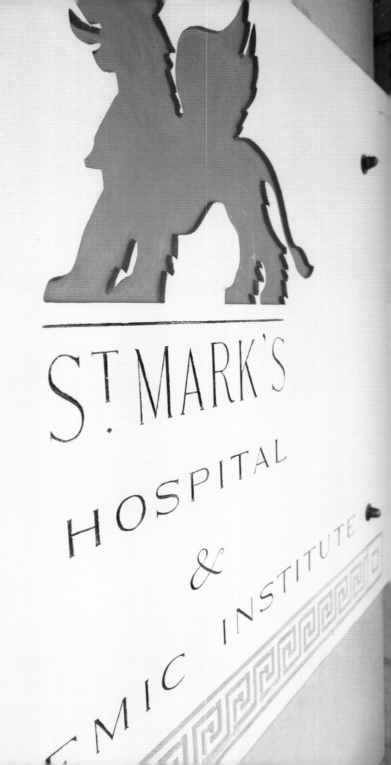

ST. MARK'S

HOSPITAL

&

EMIC INSTITUTE

Chapter 3: Ileostomy

What is an ileostomy?

An ileostomy is a stoma formed from the ileum to divert the passage of faeces (see *Fig. 3.1*). In 2006 there were nearly 6000 temporary ileostomies and about 3000 permanent ileostomies formed (IMS 2007) and there are still about 9000 ileostomies formed each year.

In appearance the ileostomy is pink or red and to touch it is warm and moist. The ileostomy is usually round or egg-shaped and it is ideally formed with a small spout of about 25 mm. The output from an ileostomy is faeces which are looser than that passed from the rectum or colostomy.

An ileostomy is active often throughout the day passing flatus and loose faeces. The output is usually about 300–900 ml daily, so it is collected in a drainable appliance that needs to be emptied four to six times daily and sometimes at night.

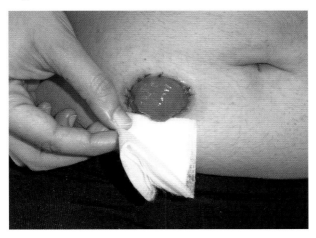

Fig. 3.1: ileostomy

Why is an ileostomy formed?

There are a variety of reasons that an ileostomy might need to be formed. They include inflammatory bowel disease such as ulcerative colitis or Crohn's disease. Furthermore people with a rectal cancer may require temporary ileostomy formation to enable the join (anastomosis) to heal.

Operations that may require an ileostomy formation

There are many operations that may result in the formation of a temporary or permanent ileostomy. The operations include a panproctocolectomy, colectomy, ileo-anal pouch and anterior resection.

Panproctocolectomy

A permanent ileostomy will be formed following an operation termed a panproctocolectomy (see *Fig. 3.2*). 'Pan-' means all or entire, 'procto-' means rectum, 'col-' relates to the colon and '-ectomy' means removal; thus it can be seen that this operation involves removing the entire rectum, colon and anus, resulting in a permanent end ileostomy. This operation has been performed for over 60 years and may be undertaken for a person with ulcerative colitis or Crohn's colitis, who is failing to respond to medical therapy.

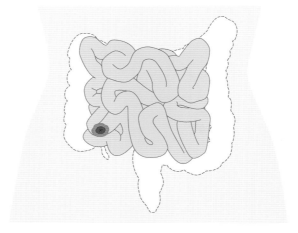

Fig. 3.2: panproctocolectomy

Colectomy

A temporary ileostomy can be formed in a variety of ways. One operation is a total colectomy or subtotal colectomy (see *Fig. 3.3*), where all or most of the colon is removed and the end of the ileum is used to form a temporary end ileostomy. As the rectum is retained it is possible to undertake further surgery to get rid of the ileostomy. This operation may be undertaken for an acutely ill person with ulcerative colitis where medicine is not resolving symptoms.

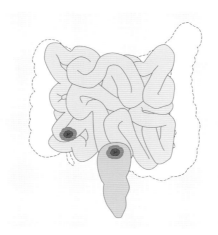

Fig. 3.3: subtotal colectomy

Ileo-anal pouch

Another operation that is used for people with ulcerative colitis that is failing to respond to medical treatment is a temporary ileostomy that will eventually result in the bowel continuity being restored, albeit differently than before. This operation is a restorative proctocolectomy, also termed a J-pouch, IPAA (ileal pouch anal anastomosis) or 'a pouch' (see *Fig. 3.4*).

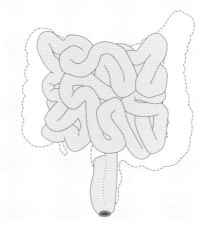

Fig. 3.4: restorative proctocolectomy

This operation can be formed in one, two or three stages. A one stage pouch is rarely performed but if it is, the colon and rectum are removed but the anal canal is retained. The end of the ileum is then formed into a new rectum, the pouch, which is anastomosed (joined) to the anal canal. A two stage pouch is the same as the one stage but then there is also a temporary loop ileostomy formed. The second stage is reversal of the loop ileostomy. A three stage pouch is a total or subtotal colectomy with a temporary end ileostomy, the second stage is removal of the rectum, formation of the pouch and a temporary loop ileostomy is formed. Finally the third and last stage is the reversal of the loop ileostomy.

Anterior resection

An anterior resection may result in the formation of a temporary loop ileostomy. This operation is undertaken for a rectal cancer that requires removal. An anterior resection is removal of part or most of the rectum and the two ends are re-joined (see *Fig. 3.5*), to maintain intestinal continuity.

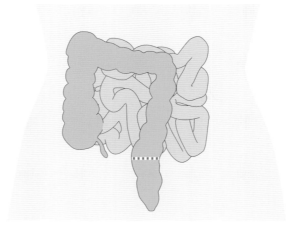

Fig. 3.5: anterior resection

This operation may not require the formation of an ileostomy to protect the healing rectum. If an ileostomy is formed during an anterior resection, when the ileostomy is reversed (closed) the passage of faeces will return to being expelled via the anus. There is a variation of this operation that is undertaken for mid or low rectal cancers called total mesorectal excision (TME). This anterior resection also includes removal of the area around the rectum which contains the blood and lymph supply and is called the mesorectum. The mesorectum is also removed because if a rectal cancer spreads it is likely to spread locally into the bowel wall or via the nearest blood supply and lymphatic drainage, so to improve the chances of removing all the cancer the mesorectum is also removed. This kind of operation is technically difficult to perform so many surgeons choose to routinely perform a loop ileostomy as there is a higher risk of an anastomotic leak occurring with a TME rather than a high anterior resection.

How is an ileostomy formed?

It is possible to form an ileostomy (and whatever operation it is formed in conjunction with) as either a laparotomy or laparoscopically. The use of laparoscopic (keyhole) surgery for all planned operations is encouraged, but there are situations where this is not possible.

An end ileostomy is formed by passing the ileum though a small incision in the abdominal wall; this is usually the diameter of two fingers. The edges of the bowel are everted, like turning over a sock top, and stitched in place. The modern spouted ileostomy was devised over 60 years ago by Bryan Brooke, to try and keep the ileostomy output away from the skin to avoid skin breakdown.

A loop ileostomy is also similarly formed, but instead of the end of the ileum being passed through the abdominal wall, a loop of small bowel is used. The bowel is partly opened, so that there are two ends visible and both are stitched onto the abdominal wall. The sutures that are used to join the bowel to the abdominal wall are dissolvable and will generally fall out six to eight weeks after the stoma is formed.

Ileostomy appliances

A standard ileostomy appliance is drainable and fastened with a Velcro-type fastening (see *Fig. 3.6*). Older types of appliance may be fastened with a plastic clip or a soft tie. There are many different ways that the appliance may be sealed and thus if there are manual dexterity issues there should be an appliance to suit each individual.

The appliance is drainable to allow drainage of the loose faeces and flatus that pass from the ileostomy to be emptied regularly throughout the day and possibly also during the night. The average change of the appliance is between once daily and every three days; this may be much longer in

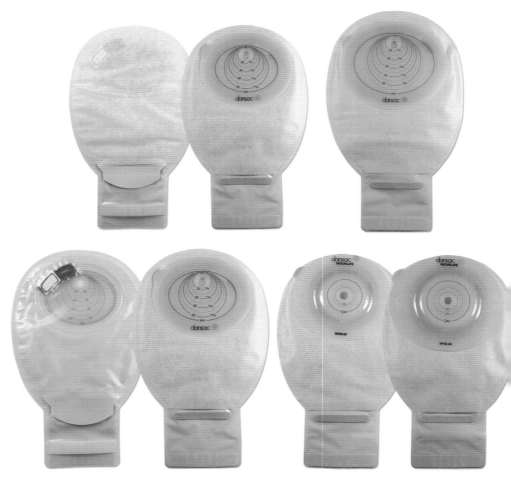

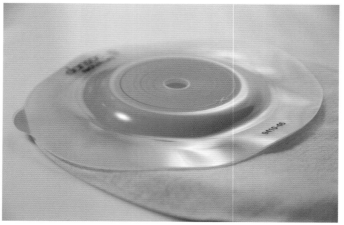

Fig. 3.6: ileostomy appliances

countries where the appliances are self-funded, such as the USA. There is usually a filter to release the flatus from the ileostomy appliance and this tends to become ineffectual if the faeces touch the inside of the filter and people will often change their appliance to ensure that the flatus does not make the appliance balloon under clothing.

There are a variety of appliance sizes available, although most people use a standard size. The appliances are also clear or opaque, with a soft cover. The clear are used in the immediate postoperative period but most people in the UK choose to wear an opaque appliance in the long-term, to cover the ileostomy output.

The ileostomy appliance requires to be emptied several times daily; often four to six times and sometimes at night. It is ideal to empty the appliance when it is a third to half full so that it is not at risk of leaking if it is not possible to empty it immediately. Regular appliance emptying also means that it will be less visible under clothing if emptied prior to being overly full.

Eating with an ileostomy

There are a number of specific dietary recommendations that are related to having an ileostomy. Unless there is already high dietary sodium, it is important to take an extra teaspoon of salt each day. Also as the faecal output is looser than a normal bowel motion, many people with an ileostomy choose to have a low residue diet and substitute brown foods for white such as white rice, bread and pasta in place of brown and wholemeal versions. Gelatin based foods such as jelly, marshmallows and wine gums also thicken the ileostomy output.

There is evidence that eating three marshmallows three times daily can reduce the average output from an ileostomy by 75 ml daily and it also thickens the output (Clarebrough et al 2015). The former helps to reduce the risk of dehydration and the latter helps to reduce the risk of an appliance leak. Furthermore to prevent dehydration it is important to drink adequate volumes of fluid without this being excessive. It is usually accepted that about two litres of non-alcoholic fluids daily are sufficient. Although, in line with government guidelines it is possible to drink alcohol, many people with an ileostomy find that beer increases the ileostomy output in unacceptable ways and may choose alcohol available in less volume, such as wine.

Pharmacology and the ileostomy

The most common specific medications used for people with an ileostomy are drugs to slow down the gut. The most commonly used drug is loperamide hydrochloride (Chandler and Lowther 2013). The dose taken by each patient can vary dramatically; some people just need one tablet a day while others require the maximum dose and some people require no medication at all. For best effect the medication should be taken 30–60 minutes prior to meals with a small drink. For people with a much higher than usual ileostomy output the additional advice is not to drink after taking the loperamide and to try and not have much fluid with the meal or for 30–60 minutes after the meal.

The patient should of course be advised to consume adequate oral fluids each day. Having an ileostomy already puts people at a risk of dehydration if adequate fluids are not consumed and it should be considered that people with an ileostomy may need to take a rehydration solution such as dioralyte, the WHO solution or the St Mark's electrolyte solution (see *Box 3.1*).

> ## Box 3.1 – St Mark's electrolyte solution
>
> - 20 g (six level 5 ml spoonsful) of glucose
> - 2.5 g (one heaped 2.5 ml spoonful) of sodium bicarbonate (baking soda)
> - 3.5 g (one level 5 ml spoonful) of sodium chloride (salt)
> - Dissolved in one litre of cold tap water

Ileostomy complications

Postoperative ileostomy needs

Sarkut et al (2015) discussed the high risk of complications associated with an ileostomy soon after surgery. When they examined who was more likely to have a problem it was men more than women and people having emergency rather than planned operations. Most of the people with ileostomy complications were successfully managed conservatively.

Dehydration

The long-term care of the ileostomy is the prevention of dehydration. Hendren et al (2015) consider that dehydration is a major cause of morbidity for people with a loop ileostomy and that it affects up to 30% of patients, resulting in the biggest cause for readmission in this patient group (Messaris et al 2012).

To address this issue Nagle et al (2012) undertook a study to examine if a training pathway with the aim to encourage self-care in patients would reduce the rates of readmission back to hospital with dehydration.

Readmission rates for dehydration went from 16% to 0% and the total readmission rate dropped from 35% to 21% respectively. Thus it can be seen that, with adequate advice, dehydration is not inevitable for people with an ileostomy. Advice to prevent dehydration should include drinking correct volumes, adding salts and being mindful of the output from the ileostomy.

Food blockage

A complication that only tends to occur for people with an ileostomy is a blockage of the bowel caused by a collection of poorly chewed food. If foods such as tough meat or vegetables are not well-chewed they may clog together and block the passage of faeces through the bowel. If this occurs the patient will report that their stoma is not active for several hours. If the blockage does not resolve the patient might become distended and subsequently nauseated and vomit.

Before the patient becomes distended it is advisable that they stop eating and try and drink plenty to dislodge the blockage. If this occurs the ileostomy will begin to work again and the food causing the blockage might be seen in the appliance. If the patient is unable to resolve the blockage themselves they should be advised to go to hospital and will often require an intravenous infusion and a nasogastric tube.

This type of conservative management will resolve a food bolus blockage in nearly all situations. It is ideal to remind the patient to be careful of eating and maybe avoid high fibre diets for a couple of days after a blockage, as they might still be a little swollen inside.

Support groups

The main support group in the UK for people with an ileostomy is the ileostomy and internal pouch support group. This group will also support people with an internal pouch.

They have a very informative website at **www.iasupport.org**. There are many local support groups also available.

References

Chandler P and Lowther C (2013) Stoma care: the use of loperamide in ileostomy care. Gastrointestinal Nursing. 11(4): 11–12.

Clarebrough E, Guest G and Stupart D (2015) Eating marshmallows reduces ileostomy output: a randomized crossover trial. Colorectal Disease. 17(12):1100–1103.

Hendren S, Hammond K, Glasgow SC, Perry WB, Buie WD et al (2015) Clinical practice guidelines for ostomy surgery. Diseases of the Colon & Rectum. 58: 375–387.

IMS (2007) referenced as ©2007 IMS Health Incorporated or its affiliates. All rights reserved. New Stoma Patient Audit GB – August 2007.

Messaris E, Sehgal R, Deiling S et al (2012) Dehydration is the most common indication for readmission after diverting ileostomy creation. Diseases of the Colon & Rectum. 55: 175–180.

Nagle D, Pare T, Keenan E, Marcet K, Tizio S et al (2012) Ileostomy pathway virtually eliminates readmissions for dehydration in new ostomates. Diseases of the Colon & Rectum. 55(12): 1266–1272.

Sarkut P, Dundar HZ, Tirnova I, Ozturk E and Yilmazlar T (2015) Is stoma care effective in terms of morbidity in complicated ileostomies? International Journal of General Medicine. 8 243–246.

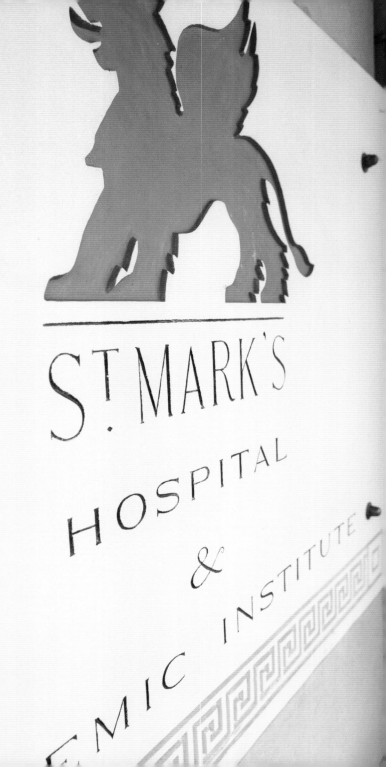

St. MARK'S

HOSPITAL

&

EMIC INSTITUTE

Chapter 4: Urinary diversion

What is a urostomy?

A urostomy, also termed an ileal conduit, is a urine output stoma (*Fig. 4.1*). A urostomy is formed when the bladder needs to be removed and the urine drained from the body in a different manner. It is estimated that there are about 11000 people in the UK with a urostomy (Nazarko 2014). The general trend, however, is a reduction in urostomy formation: in 2001 there were about 2000 new urostomies formed, five years later this had reduced to about 1500 (IMS 2007) and it is now believed that there are about 800 new urostomies formed each year (Urostomy Association 2016).

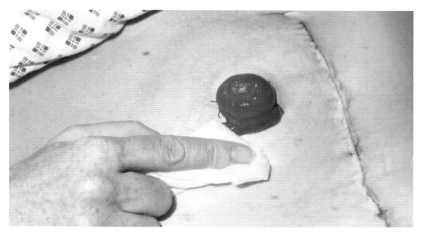

Fig. 4.1: urine output stoma

In appearance, a urostomy is pink or red and to the touch it is warm and moist; there should be a small spout of about 25 mm. The urostomy can vary, but it is generally round in shape and about 30 mm in diameter. The urostomy will generally be positioned in the right iliac fossa. The output will be urine with a little mucus and should be about 1000–2000 ml daily depending upon fluid intake and the size of the patient. The urine needs to be emptied from the urostomy appliance four to six times daily. Many people with a urostomy choose to use a leg bag or a night bag to collect urine overnight.

Why is a urostomy formed?

There are a number of reasons that a urostomy might be formed. The most common is for a bladder cancer. Other reasons include multiple sclerosis, cerebral palsy, spinal injury, interstitial cystitis, severe urinary incontinence, congenital abnormalities such as bladder extrophy and spina bifida. Multiple sclerosis (MS) is a condition that can affect the brain and/or spinal cord and may result in a variety of symptoms that can include bladder control issues. Cerebral palsy is a neurological condition that affects movement and coordination and can cause urinary incontinence. Interstitial cystitis is not well understood but presents with problems with urination and pelvic pain. Norus et al (2013) considered that in this situation many people can be successfully cured of symptoms by formation of a urostomy without the bladder being resected. Bladder extrophy is where a baby is born with the bladder protruding through the abdominal wall. Spina bifida is a condition where the spine does not develop correctly; disruption of the spinal cord and the associated nerves can result in dysfunction of the bladder or bowel.

What operations result in a urostomy formation?

Removal of the bladder, termed a cystectomy, will necessitate the formation of a urinary diversion, such as a urostomy. There are other types of internal urinary diversion that do not require a urostomy appliance.

Urinary diversions

There are a variety of urinary diversion operations available including a cystoplasty, a neobladder, a Mitrofanoff procedure, the Mainz Sigma II and an ileal conduit. Currently the neobladder is more commonly undertaken than a urostomy formation for patients that are suitable for the procedure (Herdiman et al 2013). Gerharz (2007) reviewed the published literature and considered that there was inadequate evidence to support the 'best' surgical approach, stating that each method had advantages, disadvantages and specific indications. There are no statistical differences in complication rates between people undergoing a neobladder or a urostomy formation, although people with a neobladder are more likely to experience infectious complications and the urostomy patients have more wound problems (Abe et al 2013).

Some urology procedures have in the main been superseded. These operations include bringing the ureters directly to the surface of the abdominal skin (cutaneous ureterostomy), bringing the kidney pelvis to the abdominal skin surface (cutaneous pyelostomy) or bringing the bladder through to the skin (cutaneous vesicostomy) (Harvey 1997). In addition, a colonic conduit might be formed, where a segment of the colon is used to form the conduit, but this is far less common than using the ileum.

Mitrofanoff procedure

The Mitrofanoff procedure is a surgical technique where a continent channel is created, often using the appendix. This channel is formed, creating a small continent stoma. The thin channel has an abdominal opening one end and an opening into the bladder or urinary reservoir at the other end, with continence maintained by a non-return valve in the channel. If the bladder requires removal, a Mitrofanoff procedure can still be formed in conjunction with a neobladder. To empty the bladder it is necessary to perform intermittent self-catheterisation every four to six hours (Fillingham and Douglas 2004). Thus it can be seen that careful patient selection is essential as the Mitrofanoff procedure requires patient motivation and manual dexterity to make it successful.

Cystoplasty

A cystoplasty involves replacing part or the whole of the bladder with a section of bowel. There are variations of a cystoplasty, generally related to the part of the bowel used to form it. If the whole bladder is removed and replaced this is termed a neobladder.

Neobladder

A neobladder is the formation of a new bladder using a segment of bowel. A neobladder requires a 45–70 cm section of ileum (or colon) to form the pouch or reservoir (Herdiman et al 2013). The ureters are disconnected from the bladder, which is removed, and re-implanted into the neobladder. The new reservoir is then connected to the urethra. As bowel is used there will be mucus production in the neobladder, necessitating bladder washouts in the postoperative period. A neobladder may not be possible if there is a history of bowel disease, radiotherapy or tumour that has invaded the urethra. Careful patient selection is also essential prior to formation of a neobladder, as motivation is required, for example to undertake pelvic floor exercises that are necessary to ensure that the neobladder functions well. Once urinary catheters are removed the neobladder requires retraining, although about 10% of people will have to self-catheterise intermittently in the long-term (Asgari et al 2013a).

Mainz Sigma II

Another urinary diversion is the Mainz Sigma II, where urine is diverted into the colon (which is given a pouch configuration to create a reservoir) and is then passed via the anus with the faeces (Fisch et al 1996). It was first described over 150 years ago and is not without complication, but an advantage over the formation of a urostomy is that there is no need to wear a urostomy appliance. Careful patient selection is necessary as are well functioning anal sphincter muscles. There are more complications associated with this type of urinary diversion (Nitkunan et al 2004) but it is popular in countries were the cost of stoma appliances is an issue. It is also essential to understand that the combination of faeces and urine is malodorous.

How is a urostomy formed?

It is possible to undertake a cystectomy by open, laparoscopic or robotic surgery. Robotic radical cystectomy is being increasingly performed for bladder cancer therapy, while open cystectomy is the current gold standard (Shabsigh et al 2009).

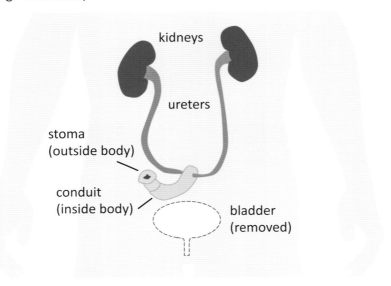

Fig. 4.2: ileal conduit or urostomy

An ileal conduit, also termed a urostomy, was first described over 60 years ago. To form a urostomy a small segment of bowel about 10–20 cm (Leach

2015; Nazaro 2014), most commonly the ileum, is surgically used to form the stoma (see *Fig. 4.2*).

It is possible to form a colonic conduit, but this is uncommon. The segment of bowel is isolated from the rest of the ileum but the blood supply is retained. The remaining parts of the ileum are rejoined (anastomosed) so that faeces are passed from the anus in the usual manner. It should be noted that because of the use of the ileum during surgery it is possible in the postoperative period that bowel function can initially be slow to return. The isolated segment of bowel is then used as a conduit (passage or channel) for the urine to pass from the ureters through the abdominal wall and to be collected within a urostomy appliance. When the urostomy is formed, one end of the ileum is sealed and the two ureters are anastomosed to it.

As ureters are very fine tubes there is a concern about this anastomosis stenosing so the urologist will use stents, inserted through the stoma and into the ureter to prevent this complication occurring in the postoperative period. The other end of the conduit is used to form the urostomy, passing through all the layers of the abdominal wall. A urostomy is a permanent, end stoma. The sutures used to join the bowel to the abdominal wall are dissolvable and take a few weeks (usually six to eight) to fall out. The bowel and the abdominal wall have usually healed for some time prior to this occurring, as there is generally superficial healing within a week of the stoma being formed.

Urostomy appliances

All urostomy appliances are drainable and fastened with a tap or bung (see *Fig. 4.3*) to enable drainage of the urine at regular times throughout the day. For people with dexterity issues there are a variety of taps or bungs available to suit the individual. To prevent the back flow of urine there is a non-return reflux inner lining incorporated within the urostomy appliance, helping to prevent urinary tract infections (Kirkwood 2006).

It is anticipated that the urostomy appliance (also termed a pouch), will be emptied about four to six times each day (Lee 2001), when it is a third to half full to ensure that the appliance does not overfill. The appliance has a maximum capacity of about 350–400 ml (Fillingham 1997) but should not be allowed to fill completely as there is the risk of the appliance leaking or showing under clothing as a bulge.

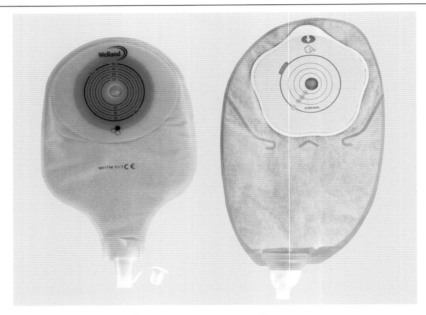

Fig. 4.3: urostomy appliances

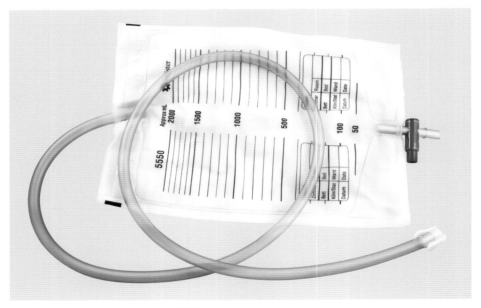

Fig. 4.4: 2000ml overnight drainage bag

The urostomy appliance should be changed every day or two, but can be left in situ for longer, particularly in countries where urostomy appliances need to be paid for.

Some people prefer to change the appliance on a daily basis as they experience a build-up of mucus within the appliance. It is important to carefully position the urostomy appliance as the tap or bung can be bulky and can become uncomfortable if not well situated. Some people prefer to wear a two-piece appliance as the angle of the bag part of the appliance can then be altered. The appliance can then be worn with the bag downwards during the day and to the side at night. This allows the urine to drain away from the urostomy appliance when attached to the night drainage bag. Some people also choose to use a leg bag if they are travelling, as this will increase the urine storage capacity. As urine production does not cease overnight, most people with a urostomy choose to wear a night drainage appliance to provide greater storage capacity of about 2000 ml (see *Fig. 4.4*). The night drainage bag can be used for one week if cleaned each day. Other alternatives include a single use night drainage bag that is disposed of daily, after the urine is emptied from the bag into the toilet.

Eating with a urostomy

In the first few days after the urostomy is formed the diet recommended is the same as for someone having undergone a bowel resection.

Many people are able to drink the same day as the stoma is formed and eat the following day. It is advocated that a light diet with small frequent meals is better tolerated in the postoperative period but there is limited evidence except for anecdote to confirm this.

There is no special diet that is necessary in the long-term with a urostomy; it is advocated that guidance on a healthy diet should be followed. It is important to keep well hydrated at all times with a urostomy. This means consuming about two to three litres daily of non-alcoholic beverages. There is no reason that alcohol cannot be safely consumed but in moderation, in line with government advice.

Specific care needs for a person with a urostomy

There is care that is only related to the urostomy, such as specific preoperative and postoperative care needs. This will be discussed in this section. Generic information on stomas is discussed elsewhere.

Specific preoperative urostomy care

Historically, all patients undergoing a urostomy formation had preoperative bowel preparation, to clear the bowel, but there are several studies that show that this is not necessary or beneficial (Tabibi et al 2007; Xu et al 2010). Due to the reduced length of stay in hospital Kristensen et al (2013) consider that preoperative training on the care of the urostomy is of benefit to patients learning how to become self-caring with their stoma.

Urostomy specific postoperative needs

To assist the bowel to function faster in the postoperative period for both flatus and faeces there is some evidence that chewing gum can be effective (Choi et al 2011); also possibly the use of an oral laxative.

In addition to the usual postoperative care it is essential for nurses to be vigilant on certain points. The specific needs for a person with a newly formed urostomy are that it should be active immediately after formation, passing urine, which might initially be blood stained. It is important to check the urine output each hour for volume, colour and the presence of urinary stents and mucus.

The urine output should be about 30 ml per hour but this will depend upon the person's age and weight. Any blood passed in the urine should quickly cease to be seen and the volume of mucus should also reduce, but mucus will always be present as the bowel conduit produces the mucus. It is important to check that the stents do not become blocked; if this is noted the stents can be gently flushed with saline (Fillingham and Douglas 2004). If a stent falls out prior to the planned removal date it should not be reinserted, but the surgeon should be advised so that they can more closely observe for an anastomotic leak. The nurse should also be vigilant for abdominal pain or tenderness and the volume of urine reducing when a stent is removed, either intentionally or accidentally.

It can be advisable to change the urostomy appliance first thing in the morning. This is ideally prior to drinking or eating to ensure that the flow of urine from the urostomy is at its lowest. This will make the appliance change simpler, as there will be less chance of urine being passed during the procedure.

Urostomy stents

The urostomy stents that are inserted during surgery are fine bore catheters, used to prevent stenosis of the anastomosis. Historically the stents were left in situ for up to two weeks. Mattei et al (2008) report on stent removal between 5–10 days postoperatively.

More recently Leach (2015) examined stent removal with specialist colleagues and concluded that if patients are clinically well and there were no intra-operative complications when anastomosing the ureters, stents could be removed between five and seven days after surgery. These early stent removal times may well not apply for people who have had pelvic radiotherapy; in this situation the stents may need to be kept in for a longer period due to the increased risk of poor healing.

When the stents are ready to be removed the nurse can gently turn the stent to help the process; alternatively a gentle pull might be necessary. Some stents, although fastened with dissolvable sutures, are not easily removed, if this occurs the nurse should give a gentle turn each day until they do fall out.

Long-term urostomy care

There are issues in the long-term that can affect a person with a urostomy.

The bowel conduit makes mucus; this is meant to assist the passage of faeces through the gastrointestinal tract. The bowel will continue to produce mucus and the person with a urostomy needs to be advised that this is normal.

Although the volume of the mucus produced and passed from the urostomy should decrease after the initial period following surgery, there will always be some mucus present in the urine. It is however important to monitor the mucus production. If this increases it can be an indication of a urine infection. Furthermore if there is a urinary infection it is usually associated with malodorous urine.

There may be changes in the odour of urine associated with foods such as oily fish, garlic, some spices, onions and asparagus. It is important for patients to know that the odour of urine can change so this is not mistaken for a urinary tract infection. There may be changes in the colour of urine with foods such as beetroot which may change it to pink or red if eaten in excess (Watson 1987). It is important to advise people with a urostomy that these transient changes in odour or colour are not a problem, nor should such foods be avoided unless the effects are bothersome.

Urostomy complications

There are several studies that discuss the complications associated specifically with urostomy formation, with the complication rates ranging from 15–64% (Kouba et al 2007; Shabsigh et al 2009; Wood et al 2003). These complications include urinary tract infections, parastomal herniation, stomal problems and renal function deterioration. It should be noted that complication rates are similar to the rates of other urinary diversions (Greenwell et al 2001; Kim et al 2014; Suzer et al 1997). Asgari et al (2013a) describe at three months after urostomy formation that nearly half of their patients had problems with managing their stoma. Despite these issues, 81% would choose again to have a urostomy compared to another urinary diversion option. In longer term studies, Maidaa et al (2014) report that the most common problems more than fifteen years after urostomy formation were related to the urostomy (49%), infections (31%), renal function (30%) and bowel function (19%).

Urinary infection

One of the most common complications associated with a urostomy is a urine infection (Mahoney et al 2013). There are many bacteria that live in the gut, increasing the risk of a urinary infection after the formation of a urostomy. To prevent a urinary infection from occurring it is advised that drinking about two to three litres daily (Blackley 1998) will maintain urine flow and thus prevent urinary stasis (Fillingham 2008); more fluids are required during hot weather and periods of exercising. As a section of bowel is used to form the urostomy, there will be small amounts of Escherichia coli (E-coli) found when the urine is tested. When undertaking a urinary dipstick test from a urostomy there will generally be a positive result for leukocytes and nitrites. Antibiotics should only be instigated if the person is symptomatic. Symptoms of a urinary tract infection include loin pain, pyrexia, feeling feverish, rigours, vomiting and the urine will appear cloudy and malodorous (Fillingham 2005).

The consumption of 250 ml of cranberry juice twice daily might be recommended to prevent a urinary infection in people with a urostomy, as it is thought to stop bacteria adhering to the wall of the conduit (Busuttil-Leaver 2004). It is also thought that cranberry juice can breakdown the mucus. Gray (2002) reports mixed results with cranberry consumption and suggests research does not prove a benefit but he does suggest that stoma specialist nurses may consider recommending regular supplementation with cranberry. In general the consumption of cranberry products is not likely to cause adverse reactions, although they are contraindicated in people taking warfarin (Suvarna et al 2003) and diabetics should use low sugar preparations.

Adding a few drops of vinegar to the urostomy bag can reduce the odour of infected urine (Lawson 2003). In the early postoperative days, additional vitamin C (Ascorbic acid 100 mg daily) can reduce mucus production. Two-piece appliances can be beneficial if mucus blocks the non-return valve, so that the pouch can be replaced on a daily basis without causing skin trauma.

Stenosis of the urostomy may result in recurrent urine infections. Treatment may involve daily dilation of the urostomy with a specialised stoma dilator (Taylor 2001). It is advisable to start with a small size and increase in diameter gradually. Dilators should be used with care, as splitting the skin can cause further scarring. If dilation is ineffective surgery may be required (Taylor 1999).

Taking a sample from a urostomy

A urinary specimen should not be taken from the urostomy appliance for testing. A sample should be taken via the urostomy with a single use catheter, using an aseptic technique. Mahoney et al (2013) suggest that although the stoma should be cleaned with sterile gauze prior to taking the sample it is uncertain if this should be in conjunction with soap and water, sterile water, normal saline, povidone-iodine or chlorhexidine. The gauze should be used to clean from the centre of the stoma outwards and the stoma should be blotted dry. They consider a large catheter diameter such as a 16Fr should be used to allow mucus to pass. The open end of the catheter should be inserted into the specimen pot and then the catheter should be gently inserted a few centimetres (3–7 cm) into the urostomy (Dougherty and Lister 2015). If resistance is felt on insertion, the catheter should be gently rotated but not forced. The drops of urine can then be collected into a sterile urine specimen pot; about 5–10 ml is required. It should be noted that it can take a few minutes to collect. The catheter should be discarded after use and the urostomy appliance replaced. If this is not possible, it is acceptable to collect drops from the cleaned urostomy directly into a sterile specimen pot.

Urine crystal formation

Due to the alkaline urine there may be the formation of oxalate crystals (phosphate deposits) on or around the urostomy (Lawson 2003). These crystals may cause irritation, bleeding or possibly ulceration to the urostomy (Leaver 1996). White vinegar can be diluted, in equal proportions with water, and used to dissolve the crystals by direct application to the stoma. Cranberry juice can then be drunk regularly to try and restore the pH level and thus reduce the subsequent formation of crystals (Fillingham 2005).

Sexual issues with a urostomy

Formation of a urostomy is associated with sexual difficulties that include erectile dysfunction and ejaculatory problems with all of the respondents in one study reporting sexual problems (Pazar et al 2015), whereas Asgari et al (2013b) report that after a period of twelve months recuperation, 10% of the men that were able to undertake sexual intercourse prior to their operation were able to after the formation of their urostomy. They report that although their spouses were accepting of the urostomy it nonetheless negatively affected their relationship. Asgari et al (2013a) reported that the rates of erectile dysfunction was about the same for men with a urostomy, neobladder or Mainz pouch. In women there may be dyspareunia for several months after surgery (Herdiman et al 2013).

Support groups

The national support group in the UK for people with a urostomy is the Urostomy Association (UA), initially formed in 1971 as the Urinary Conduit Association, changing to its current name in 1984. The association has an informative website at **urostomyassociation.org.uk**. There are many local support groups also available.

References

Abe T, Takada N, Shinohara N, Sazawa A, Maruyama S et al (2013) A comparison of 90–day complications between ileal conduit and neobladder reconstruction after radical cystectomy: a multi-institutional retrospective study in Japan. The Journal of Urology. 1894S: e216.

Asgari MA, Safarinejad MR, Shakhssalim N, Soleimani M, Shahabi A et al (2013a) Quality of life after radical cystectomy for bladder cancer in men with an ileal conduit or continent urinary diversion: A comparative study. Annals of Urology. 5(3): 190–196.

Asgari MA, Safarinejad MR, Shakhssalim N, Soleimani M, Shahabi A et al (2013b) Sexual function after non nerve-sparing radical cystoprostatectomy: a comparison between ileal conduit urinary diversion and orthotopic ileal neobladder substation. Internatinal Brazilian Journal of Urology. 39(4): 474–483.

Black P (2000) Holistic stoma care. Baillière Tindall. London.

Blackley P (1998) Practical stoma wound and continence management. Research Publications Pty Ltd. Victoria, Australia.

Busutil-Leaver R (2004) Reconstructive surgery for the promotion of continence. In: Fillingham S and Douglas J (eds) Urological nursing. 3rd ed. Churchill Livingstone. Edinburgh.

Choi H, Kang SH, Yoon DK, Kang SG, Ko HY et al (2011) Chewing gum has timulatory effect on bowel motility in patients after open or robotic radical cystectomy for bladder cancer: a prospective randomized comparative study. Urology. 77(4): 884–890.

Dougherty L and Lister S (2015) The Royal Marsden manual of clinical nursing procedures. 9th edition. Wiley-Blackwell. West Sussex.

Fillingham S (2008) Urinary diversion. In: Burch J (ed) Stoma care. Wiley-Blackwell. West Sussex.

Fillingham S (2005) Care of patients with urological stomas. In: Breckman B (ed) Stoma care and rehabilitation. Elsevier Churchill Livingstone. Edinburgh.

Fillingham S and Douglas J (2004) Urological nursing. 3rd ed. Churchill Livingstone. Edinburgh.

Fillingham S (1997) Urological stomas. In: Fillingham S and Douglas J (eds.) Urological Nursing. 2nd ed. Baillière Tindall. London.

Fisch M, Wammack R and Hohenfeller R (1996) The sigma rectum pouch (Mainz pouch II). World Journal of Urology 14: 68–72.

Gerharz EW (2007) is there any evidence that one continent diversion is any better than any other or than ileal conduit? Current Opinions in Urology. 17: 402–407.

Gray M (2002) Are cranberry juice and cranberry products effective in the prevention or management of urinary tract infection. Journal of Wound Ostomy and Continence Nursing. 29(3): 122–6.

Greenwell T, Venn SN and Mundy AR (2001) Review: Augmentation cystoplasty. British Journal of Urology International. 88(6): 511–525.

Harvey H (1997) Urological stomas. In: Fillingham, S. and Douglas, J. (eds) Urological Nursing. Baillière Tindall. London.

Herdiman O, Ong K, Johnson L and Lawrentschuk N (2013) Orthotopic bladder substitution (neobladder): Part II: Postoperative complications, management and long-term follow-up. Journal of Wound Ostomy and Continence Nursing. 40(2): 171–180.

IMS (2007) referenced as ©2007 IMS Health Incorporated or its affiliates. All rights reserved. New Stoma Patient Audit GB – August 2007.

Kim SH, Yu A, Jung JH, Lee YJ and Lee ES (2014) Incidence and risk factors of 30–Day early and 90–day late morbidity and mortality of radical cystectomy during a 13–year follow-up: a comparative propensity-score matched analysis of complications between neobladder and ileal conduit. Japanese Journal of Clinical Oncology. 44(7): 677–685.

Kirkwood L (2006) An introduction to stomas. Journal of Community Nursing. 19(7): 20–25.

Kouba E, Sands M, Lentz A, Wallen E and Pruthi RS (2007) A comparison of the Bricker versus Wallace ureteroileal anastomosis in patients undergoing urinary diversion for bladder cancer. Journal of Urology. 178(3): 945–9.

Kristensen SA, Laustsen S, Kiesbye B and Jensen BT (2013) The urostomy education scale: a reliable and valid tool to evaluate urostomy self-care skills among cystectomy patients. Journal of Wound Ostomy and Continence Nursing. 40(6): 611–617.

Lawson A (2003) Complications of stomas. In Elcoat C (ed) Stoma care nursing. Hollister. London.

Leach D (2015) Ureteric stent removal post cycstectomy. British Journal of Nursing. 24(22): S20–S26.

Leaver RB (1996) Cranberry juice. Professional Nurse. 11(8): 525–526.

Lee J (2001) Common stoma problems: a brief guide for community nurses. British Journal of Community Nursing. 6(8): 407–413.

Maidaa M, Miranda G, Gill I, Schuckman A, Daneshmand S et al (2014) Long-term clinical outcome and complications after radical cystectomy and ileal conduit. The Journal of Urology. 191(4S): e82.

Mattei A, Birkhaeuser FD, Baermann C, Warncke SH and Studer UE (2008) To stent or not to stent pre-operatively the ureteroileal anastomosis of ileal orthotopic bladder substitutes and ileal conduits? Results of a prospective randomized trial.

The Journal of Urology. 179(2): 582–586.

Mahoney M, Baxter K, Burgess J, Bauer C, Downey C et al (2013) Procedure for obtaining a urine sample from a urostomy, ileal conduit, and colon conduit a best practice guideline for clinicians. Journal of Wound, Ostomy and Continence Nursing. 40(3): 277–279.

Nazaro L (2014) Urostomy management in the community. British Journal of Community Nursing. 19(9): 448–452.

Nitkunan T, Leaver R, Patel HR and Woodhouse CR (2004) Modified ureterosigmoidostomy (Mainz II): a long-term follow-up. British Journal of Urology International. 93(7): 1043–1047.

Norus T, Fode M and Norling J (2013) Ileal conduit without cystectomy may be an appropriate option in the treatment of intractable bladder pain syndrome/interstitial cystitis. The Journal of Urology. 189(4S): e357.

Pazar B, Yava A and Başal Ş (2015) Health-related quality of life in persons living with a urostomy. Journal of Wound Ostomy and Continence Nursing. 42(3): 264–270.

Shabsigh A, Korets R, Vora KC, Brooks CM, Cronin AM et al (2009) Defining early morbidity of radical cystectomy for patients with bladder cancer using a standardized reporting methodology. European Urology. 55(1): 164–174.

Suvarna R, Pirmohamed M and Henderson L (2003) Possible interaction between warfarin and cranberry juice. British Medical Journal. 327(7429): 1454.

Suzer O, Vates TS, Freedman AL, Smith CA and Gonzales R (1997) Results of the Mitrofanoff procedure in urinary tract reconstruction in children. British Journal of Urology International. 79(2): 279–282.

Tabibi A, Simforoosh N, Basiri A, Ezzatnejad M, Abdi H et al (2007) Bowel preparation versus no preparation before ileal urinary diversion. Urology. 70(4): 654–658.

Taylor P (2001) Care of patients with complications following formation of a stoma. Professional Nurse. 17(4): 252–254.

Taylor P (1999) Stomal complications. In Taylor P (ed) Stoma care in the community: A clinical resource for practitioners. NT books. London. https://urostomyassociation. org.uk/information/urostomy/ accessed 26 May 2016.

Watson D (1987) Drug therapy – colour changes to faeces and urine. Pharmaceutical Journal 236: 68.

Wood DN, Allen S, Greenwell TJ and Shah PJR (2003) Stomal complications of ileal conduit diversion. British Journal of Urology. 91(supplement 2): 92.

Xu R, Zhao X, Zhong Z, Zhang L (2010) No advantage is gained by preoperative bowel preparation in radical cystectomy and ileal conduit: a randomized controlled trial of 86 patients. International Urology and Nephrology. 42(4): 947–950.

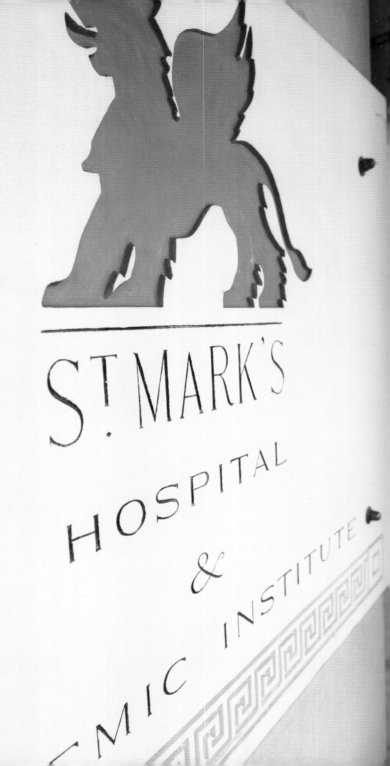

Chapter 5: Other issues

Stoma complications

There are many different complications associated with having a stoma formed. The most common is sore skin around the stoma. In a UK audit by Cottam and Richards (2006) of nearly 4000 newly formed stomas, the short-term complications included mucosal separation (24%), necrosis (9%) and retraction (40%). When a problem is noted it is important for the nurse to undertake a full assessment of the situation, plan an appropriate intervention, implement the treatment and re-evaluate the effectiveness of the treatment.

Flatus

In an old study by Pringle and Swan (2001) three-quarters of people with a stoma reported that flatus was an issue to them. This reduced to just over half by a year after the stoma was formed, suggesting that adaptation does occur over time. Practical ways to reduce flatus include avoiding smoking, chewing gum, using drinking straws and talking while eating. Certain food also produce more wind, such as cabbage, and these can be avoided if desired.

Sore skin

There are a number of reasons that the skin around the stoma can become sore, including pre-existing skin conditions such as eczema. It is also important to consider potential causes of the sore skin such as a leaking appliance, which may be due to a stoma that is retracted, stenosed or prolapsed, causing the appliance not to adhere well. Additionally, changes in the shape of the abdominal wall can result in the appliance not adhering well. This may be due to pregnancy or weight loss, for example, and may result in a leaking appliance. Leakage from the stoma appliance causing sore skin is termed irritant contact dermatitis and Ratcliff et al (2005) reported two months after the stoma is formed that 10% of people with a stoma had sore skin for this reason.

When assessing the sore skin it is important to consider describing it, using words such as broken, oozing, bleeding and ulcerated for example. The extent of the sore skin is also important, such as whether it is close to the stoma or includes all of the skin under the flange. There are a number of assessment tools that can be used to guide the nurse to make this assessment.

Sometimes careful cleaning and drying of the peristomal skin is all that is needed, in conjunction with a correctly sized appliance aperture. If problems do not resolve within a few days the patient should be advised to see their stoma specialist nurse.

Allergy

Complications can include an allergy to the stoma products (see *Fig. 5.1*), although this is rare (Lyon and Smith 2009). Sensitivity to stoma products is more common and both problems are treated initially by changing the appliance to one from a different manufacturer. The patient can also be referred to a dermatologist if problems persist.

Mucocutaneous separation

In the immediate postoperative period the join between the skin and the stoma that is stitched together with dissolvable sutures can break down (see *Fig. 5.2*). The separation can be one small section, circumferential, shallow or deep. Treatment can be to simply regularly review the separation but with no additional change in care, or it may require stoma powder or packing (if deep). The surgeon should be informed of this complication if it occurs and it may be caused by tension on the sutures or a localised infection.

Granuloma

Red cauliflower-like nodules can occur at the edge of the stoma and are called overgranulation or granulomas (see *Fig. 5.3*). They are more common around a colostomy than an ileostomy and are often the result of friction from the stoma flange or irritation from the faeces. Treatment can be the use of silver nitrate directly on the granulomas (ASCN 2015).

Prolapsed stoma

A prolapsed stoma can be seen when the bowel intussuscepts or telescopes out and becomes longer (see *Fig. 5.4*). In some cases it can just be a little longer than a normal stoma, but in extensive cases the prolapsing bowel can fill the appliance. It is however fairly rare, with Persson et al (2005) reporting two per cent of people with an ileostomy with a prolapsed stoma. The cause can be increased abdominal pressure. Treatment can include surgical refashioning of the stoma but this is not always required.

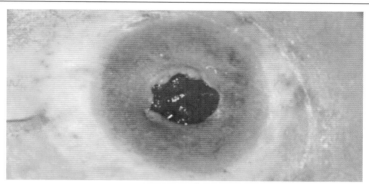

Fig. 5.1: allergies

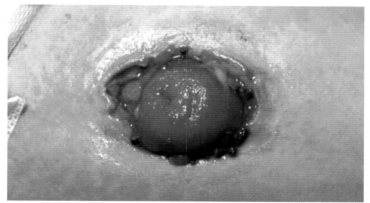

Fig. 5.2: mucotaneous separation

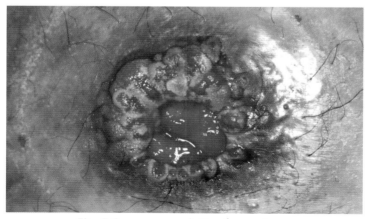

Fig. 5.3: overgranulation/granuloma

Patients should be advised to carefully check their stoma at every appliance change for signs of damage and a surgeon or stoma specialist nurse should assess the prolapse.

Stenosed stoma

A stenosed stoma can occur where the lumen of the bowel narrows and this causes problems with the stoma allowing passage of faeces or urine from the body. Persson et al (2005) report this is a problem for 7% of people with an ileostomy. Treatment can be dilation of the stoma or surgical refashioning.

Retracted stoma

A retracted stoma appears to be pulled back into the abdomen (see *Fig. 5.5 and 5.6*) and occurs in about 2% of people with a stoma (Persson et al 2005). The cause may be related to the bowel being under too much tension or weight gain. Retraction can also be the result of a necrotic stoma; after the dead tissue has been removed the remaining stoma is smaller and often retracted. Treatment will depend upon what problems result from the retraction; if it is appliance leakage the use of a convex appliance may be helpful.

Factors that affect the adherence of the flange

The appliance must be able to adhere to the peristomal skin. It is important to change the appliance regularly, or as soon as possible after a leak occurs. Thus patients are advised to keep a spare stoma appliance change kit for unexpected appliance changes when away from home.

The length of time an appliance will stay adhered to the peristomal skin depends on many things, such as the weather, skin condition, scars, body shape near the stoma and the nature of the stoma output:

- Moist, oily skin or oil applied to the peristomal skin may reduce wear-time
- Weight changes, such as weight gained or lost after surgery, can change the shape of the abdomen
- Diet may affect the seal of the appliance; a watery output is more likely to break through a seal and cause an appliance to leak than a thicker output

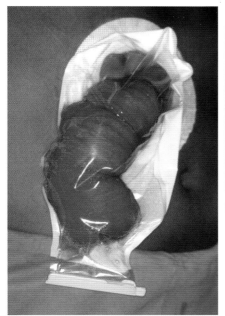

Fig. 5.4: prolapsed stoma

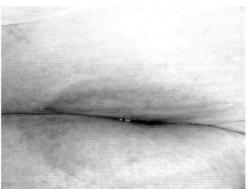

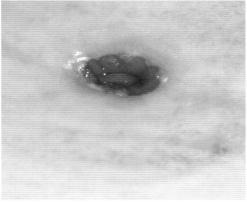

Fig. 5.5 and 5.6: retracted stomas

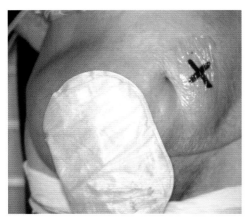

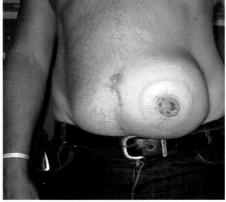

Fig. 5.7 and 5.8: parastomal hernia

- Physical activities may affect wear-time such as swimming, strenuous sports or anything that causes sweating
- Sweating: body heat added to the outside temperature can cause skin barriers to loosen more quickly than usual

If any of the above cause an issue, the person with a stoma should be advised to contact their stoma specialist nurse for advice.

Parastomal hernia

A parastomal hernia is seen as a bulging around the stoma (see *Fig. 5.7 and 5.8*) and is due to the weakness of the abdominal wall where the incision has been made to form the stoma. There is an old study that showed that wearing a support belt from three months after the stoma is formed in conjunction with abdominal exercises significantly reduced the incidence of a parastomal hernia at one year (Thompson and Trainor 2005) and at the three year follow-up (Thompson and Trainor 2007).

Rates did rise to one in five people having a hernia at three years but the authors also reported that many of the patients were no longer using their belt or performing their exercises, which might have contributed to this increased rate. Liu et al (2014) reported nearly one in three people with a urostomy had a parastomal hernia a few years after the stoma was formed. In this group, almost half had a surgical repair mainly due to abdominal pain. Cowin and Redmond (2012) consider that almost one in two people with a urostomy have a parastomal hernia.

It appears that hernia formation increases over time and is related to obesity and having a laparotomy. This further supports the need for life-long follow-up by the nurse for people who have a stoma formed.

Stoma accessories

Products to assist in the care of a stoma, often called stoma accessories (see *Fig. 5.9*), need to be carefully assessed to ensure that they are appropriately used. The cost of prescribing accessory products in England has risen from almost £13 million in 2000 to over £53 million two years later (Black 2013). It might be assumed that using more expensive stoma appliances or the use of stoma accessories will increase the cost of prescriptions; however this may not be the case (McPhail et al 2014).

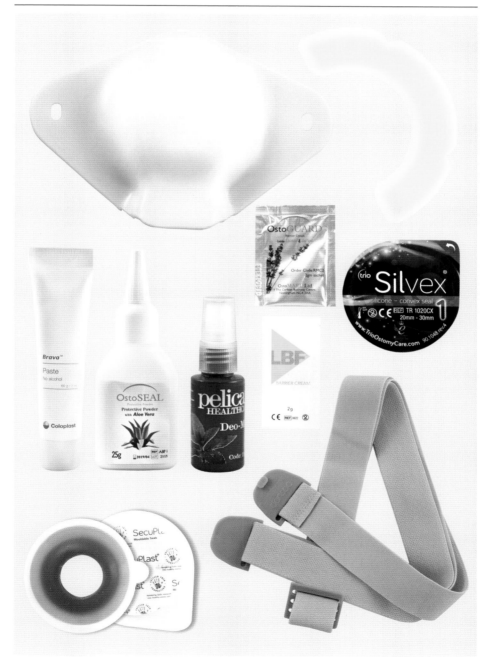

Fig. 5.9: stoma accessories

A saving will occur if an accessory reduces the number of leaking appliances and thus reduces the number of appliance changes. Therefore great care has to be taken when prescribing stoma products from a formulary; use of the cheapest products in an attempt to save money may be counterproductive. That said, products are similar in many ways and for the majority of patients most appliances will result in a good appliance seal without leaks.

When examining people with a urostomy McPhail et al (2014) reported that not everyone used anything in addition to their urostomy appliance, but the majority did. The most common accessory used (by nearly two-thirds of people) was a protective barrier wipe.

Stoma powder

Stoma powder is used on sore, wet skin. It should be used after the skin is cleaned and dried and needs to be used sparingly, with the majority dusted off or it can clog and prevent the appliance from adhering to the skin.

Protective skin barrier

There are a number of protective barriers available that come as wipes or sprays. Protective barriers are used after the skin is cleaned and dried to protect the skin from the stoma output, which can cause the skin to become sore if it is corrosive (Berry et al 2007).

Paste and seals

There are a number of seals and pastes available that are used on the skin around the stoma to fill creases or skin dips and make the skin surface more level. Paste is softer and can take a while to 'dry' so it should be used sparingly. Some paste contains alcohol so will sting if used on broken skin. Seals are more firm and can be used in their entirety or broken into smaller pieces as required.

Convex appliance

A convex flange is shaped as a dome rather than flat. Convexity can vary from soft to hard, and is used for retracted stomas or stomas that have a skin dip. A convex appliance should only be used after a careful assessment by the stoma specialist nurse. There is a risk that the pressure from the convex flange can cause a break in the skin or even ulceration. At each appliance change the skin around the stoma should be carefully examined for any signs of bruising which might be a precursor for sore skin occurring.

Chemotherapy and the stoma

Chemotherapy for a bowel or bladder cancer can have a number of associated side-effects. These are shown in *Box 5.1*. The side-effects can be reduced in severity or resolved by certain treatments. Nausea can be treated with antiemetics. Sore and numb fingers can be a problem when caring for the stoma, but symptoms often settle after treatment is completed although problems can be permanent. Changes in gut function such as loose stool can be improved by medication such as loperamide to slow down the gut transit, and by taking a low fibre diet and extra fluids. A sore mouth can be made less painful by using a soft toothbrush and mouthwash. Tiredness may be due to anaemia and if so should be treated; it might be necessary in the short-term to plan to perform tasks such as stoma appliance changes in the morning when the person has more energy and to have regular breaks to rest. Bleeding may occur if the level of the platelets is low and care should be taken when cleaning the very vascular stoma to prevent bleeding while waiting for the platelet level to resolve.

Box 5.1 - Chemotherapy side-effects

- Nausea and vomiting
- Sore hands and feet
- Numbness/tingling in the hands and feet
- Changes in the gut function
- Sore mouth
- Tiredness
- Bleeding

Radiotherapy and the stoma

After radiotherapy there can be a number of side-effects, some of which can last for many years. These side effects are summarised in *Box 5.2*. The side-effects can be reduced in severity by avoiding caffeine and alcohol. The abdominal pain may be due to the formation of abdominal adhesions inside the abdominal cavity; this pain may reduce over time. Changes in the gut function can be treated as for the chemotherapy side-effects. Urinary problems may require antibiotics to treat infections. In relation to sexual issues, there may be changes to the vagina, making it drier and with less elasticity making intercourse uncomfortable. The use of lubrication may assist in this situation. Patients can be reassured that tiredness does usually resolve within a few months of completing the radiotherapy. Skin may become drier, flaky and itchy, which may cause problems with flange adherence. The patient should be advised to contact the stoma specialist nurse to resolve any of these issues.

Box 5.2 - Radiotherapy side-effects

- Abdominal pain
- Changes in the gut function
- Urinary problems
- Sexual problems
- Tiredness
- Skin changes

Employment

Having a stoma disrupts the working life of the individual. For most people with a stoma, work can be resumed after a period of convalescence, but occasionally a job change may be necessary and this can cause a decrease in earnings. Pazar et al (2015) report many people with a urostomy had not returned to their job four months after surgery for reasons such as fear of appliance leakages. Prior to returning to work it is ideal for patients to speak to their employer and initially working fewer hours can be beneficial.

Travel

Many people who have had a stoma operation feel that they will never be able to travel or go on holiday again, while a few patients make a plan to go away as soon as they are well enough and will not let the thought of the stoma deter them. Going away on holiday and travelling once the patient is well enough takes a little bit more planning than previously, but taking time to think about what will be needed for stoma care will be advantageous. Remembering to prepare well before travelling will avoid mishaps and a discussion can take place with the stoma specialist nurse about what will be needed.

Before travelling

In the rehabilitation period after stoma surgery, small trips away from home, perhaps overnight, will help to instil confidence. This will enable patients to have assurance that their appliance is safe and that any problems can be sorted out without anxiety.

Patients should be advised to contact the stoma specialist nurse and ask for advice and discuss where they are going and what they will need to take. A travel certificate is available in several European languages that can be given to security or customs to explain about the stoma and the stoma supplies in the hand luggage. Also if travelling in Europe patients should have an up-to-date EHIC card that allows reciprocal care in a European public hospital.

Arrangement of private travel insurance is advised before travel and it is important that the policy does not exclude pre-existing conditions. For travel in the UK, a RADAR key (now called the National Key Scheme) that provides access to disabled facilities at motorways and other places, can be useful. The voluntary support organisations also provide advice about travelling with a stoma and may be able to provide contacts for travel insurance. Patients who have an appliance company who deliver their supplies can enquire if the supplier will deliver to other destinations if individuals are travelling for more than two weeks.

Flammable solvents such as adhesive remover and skin cleansers are not allowed on aeroplanes but the stoma specialist nurse or pharmacist should be able to suggest a suitable alternative. Many of the stoma delivery companies supply a travel stoma change bag that has a hook to hang on a toilet door and a mirror to help when changing the appliance whilst travelling.

It is advisable to take double the amount of appliances usually used to allow for any emergencies such as diarrhoea with change of food and water.

On the journey

When travelling it is advisable to keep all the stoma supplies in the hand luggage and not in the hold in case the hold luggage does not arrive. Ensure that enough appliances are ready-cut and prepared in case of emergency, as scissors will have to go into the hold luggage.

If the stoma has settled to a regular size, pre-cut appliances can be used. If flying it may be useful to book a seat near to the toilet and use the toilet before the meal service starts, so allowing enough time for an appliance change if needed.

Also for individuals who have any surgery to the perineal area an aisle seat is convenient as it will allow legs to be stretched and positions to be changed if the perineal area is still tender. Carbonated drinks should be avoided on aeroplanes as the change in pressure will cause added wind; eating regular meals can help to reduce flatus.

Patients who travel by car must use a seat belt at all times. If this is difficult across the abdomen and stoma, a device can be bought in a car accessory shop that can be used on inertia seat belts. The device keeps the seat belt slack until the brakes are suddenly applied and then it releases and keeps the individual braced in the seat.

Food and drink

Most hotels, other holiday accommodation and ships have en-suite facilities available, making appliance change easy. Patients travelling to hot countries and on religious pilgrimages will need to keep their appliances in a cool place to avoid the flange melting.

Care should be taken with food and drink whilst abroad; for example ice cubes and salads should be avoided as they are often made or washed in local water. Only bottled water should be drunk. Food that has been left out for a long time should be avoided and exotic food should be taken in moderation. If travelling long haul, patients should be advised to acclimatise themselves across a few days, spend only moderate amounts of time in the sun, keep up fluid levels at all times and avoid too much alcohol. It is useful to take a supply of anti-diarrhoeal medication and rehydration solutions in case of need.

Patients who irrigate their colostomy should only use bottled water whilst abroad. It is advisable for people with a colostomy to take a supply of drainable stoma appliances in case of an emergency while away, including if they usually irrigate.

On the beach

Patients who have a stoma can swim in the sea or a pool. For men who have a stoma, boxer type swimming trunks are often preferred, as they come up over the stoma site and if necessary a pair of ordinary trunks can be worn underneath.

For women a one-piece costume with a ruched abdominal area works well as does a tankini. It is advisable to change or empty the appliance before swimming and if necessary change the appliance after swimming. Appliances taken to the beach should be kept out of direct sunlight. There is swimwear for patients with stomas available online and from stoma suppliers, but often a suitable garment can be found in the high-street shops.

Stoma reversal

Closing or reversing a colostomy

If a patient has been advised that their colostomy can be reversed or closed, the surgeon might mention plans to do this in a few months when they have recovered from the first surgery. It is advisable to speak to the surgeon or stoma specialist nurse for advice. Many things must be taken into account when thinking about closing a colostomy, such as:

- The reason the person needed the colostomy in the first place
- Whether the person is suitable for more surgery
- The patient's health since the operation and any other comorbidities
- Other problems that may have come up during or after surgery
- Whether the patient wants to have their colostomy reversed

Some older patients do not want to have the colostomy reversed as they are able to manage on a day-to-day basis. Having a colostomy can make their life more tolerable or they realise reversal may mean they are incontinent of faeces.

Ileostomy closure

There is evidence that a temporary ileostomy may not be reversed in all situations. David et al (2010) report that as many as one in four are not closed and this increases to one in three if there are any other comorbidities. Interestingly only twelve per cent of reversals occur within twelve weeks of the stoma formation. This was found by Jackson and Barnwall (2014) who also report that eleven per cent of people with a stoma were not reversed. They reported that median length of time to wait for a reversal was five months. People requiring chemotherapy often waited nine months before the ileostomy was reversed. For many people, after a stoma reversal there is a temporary time when the bowel readjusts and this can be quite problematic.

Anterior resection syndrome

Anterior resection syndrome is a term used to describe symptoms experienced by people after they have had part or most of their rectum surgically removed. Symptoms include urgency and frequency, where the person needs to urgently go to the toilet to have their bowels open. Bowel frequency is as a result of a reduced storage capacity and thus more trips to the toilet are required to pass small amounts of faeces.

Some patients have difficulty with continence. These symptoms generally settle down within a few weeks of the anterior resection or within a few weeks of having the stoma reversed. If symptoms do not settle treatment options include medication such as loperamide to slow down the gut and dietary changes, such as a low fibre diet. If these simple measures fail, bowel retraining in the form of biofeedback may be necessary.

Body image

Adaptation to the changed physical body and to the psychological body image that the individual has is a complex phenomenon. Intrinsic factors, such as the individuals coping mechanisms, and extrinsic factors, such as the socio-cultural background of the community the individual comes from, will have an impact on how the individual perceives their stoma (Porrett and McGrath, 2005). Ang et al (2013) suggest that there are many factors that have a positive or negative effect on the individual's adaptation to stoma formation but psychological issues are often under-emphasised in clinical practice or unrecognised by nurses. Self and identity are in an ever-evolving process of becoming and are never thought to be complete. Individuals have cited feelings of frustration, helplessness and worry about what others will think of them. Often the biggest fears are the lack of control of odour or noise and of an appliance leakage whilst in a public place. Stoma appliance disposal can also affect the individual's psychological wellbeing and body image. Concerns about changing the stoma appliance and disposing of the used appliance can result in people avoiding social and leisure activities (McKenzie et al 2006).

Psychological distress

In assessing the psychological distress factor of having a colostomy, almost half believed that the colostomy ruled their lives. Having a stoma and changes in appearance can increase frustration and anger and also lower self-esteem, confidence and feelings of wellbeing (Krouse et al 2007). Persson et al (2005) state that the nurse education patients received was inadequate and contributed to their difficulty in adjusting.

Individuals with a stoma also report alienation, feeling shame, embarrassment, changes in quality of life, roles and relationships in their social environment. These findings suggest that more attention needs to be paid to the psychosocial needs of patients, with efforts being focussed on confronting non-adaptive coping mechanisms to enable the individual to return to their daily activities more quickly and successfully. Feelings of shock and disgust are identified in individuals when seeing the stoma for the first time and are elevated in the individuals who have not been prepared preoperatively.

Adaptation to a stoma

The transformational process that an individual goes through after the formation of a stoma requires social and psychological adjustments. However, as Notter and Burnard (2006) reveal, many individuals with a stoma, in practice, find the adaptation process difficult and never reconcile themselves to returning to their previous lifestyle.

Social isolation can manifest itself in many forms and is not confined to individuals who live alone. The socially isolated suffer worse health status, have a higher consumption of healthcare resources and may have poorer outcomes after surgery. The individual's adaptation to living with a stoma and their technical expertise with the appliance are strongly associated with their emotional, social and sexual rehabilitation. It is estimated that individuals who are depressed or anxious at ten weeks after stoma surgery are most likely to still be experiencing psychological problems a year later. The nurse is in a privileged position to guide the individual in the transition from bowel or bladder disease to health, achieved by enabling them to become autonomous in their stoma care.

Quality of life

Living with the reality of having a stoma can have a profoundly negative impact on the individual, and not everyone adjusts well. The seminal work on the role of the stoma specialist nurse was by Wade (1989) 'A Stoma is for Life'. Wade suggested that patients with a stoma specialist nurse had better outcomes than those without one. In the 1980s there were few stoma specialist nurses; now there are an estimated 650 in the UK. Furukawa et al (2013) consider that the health-related quality of life is lower for people with a urostomy when compared to other stoma types, but that over time quality of life does improve.

Sexual relations

Some individuals or couples may readily accept cessation or limitation of sexual activity after surgery, but for others this can lead to a significant crisis in their life. For some people, sexual activity can be placed on hold during the postoperative and early rehabilitation stages, dependent on the extent of the surgery (Goodhart 2011).

Disclosure of sexual problems after surgery is a sensitive issue for the patient and the nurse, but overcoming embarrassment is critical. Work by Gianotten et al (2006) suggested that there is a resistance by healthcare professionals to discussing sexual issues. This may be due to lack of knowledge or embarrassment. Borwell (2009) suggests that nurses should have a basic understanding of sexuality and use a specific framework such as the PLISSIT model of sexual health (Annon 1976). In this framework the individual may need 'permission' to explore difficult matters with the nurse; permission can be gained by the nurse bringing up the subject. The patients can discuss their concerns, such as appliance leakage during intimate moments. In the 'specific suggestions stage' the nurse provides further information in the form of written literature or referral to another healthcare professional. Here a sexual history is important for the healthcare professional or for referral onwards.

Intensive therapy may be required for some couples, to include relationship counselling as well as sexual counselling.

Sexual dysfunction, loss of sensation, reduced feelings of pleasure and actual physical inability to have sexual intercourse are common long-term consequences of pelvic cancer surgery in both men and women. The potential for sexual dysfunction should be discussed with the patient prior to surgery by both the surgeon and stoma specialist nurse. Sperm production can be affected by radiotherapy and chemotherapy and for younger males sperm banking should be discussed. Pelvic surgery such as abdominoperineal excision of the rectum may cause either transient or permanent erectile dysfunction following damage to the autonomic nerves which control the blood supply to the penis resulting in sensory loss, lack of erection and ejaculatory problems.

In females, rectal surgery may result in altered pelvic anatomy with scarring causing vaginismus, dyspareunia (Ozturk et al 2015) and penetration difficulties. Pelvic and anal irradiation may cause stenosis and dryness of the vagina and the women may need to be taught how to dilate their vagina. Likewise some chemotherapy treatments may cause vaginal infections with resultant odour and problems with self-esteem (Borwell 2009).

Ramirez et al (2009) discussed that some women felt that having a stoma would make it difficult to have a sexual partner in the belief that they 'smelt' and therefore would be undesirable. Furthermore that it would be difficult to explain to a potential partner their physical condition. Kilic et al (2007) conclude that stoma patients with a supportive partner had better self-esteem, body image and sexual communication; the latter is essential to enable the couple to discuss any difficulties.

Partners' reactions to the stoma

Stoma-forming surgery can have emotional consequences for the individual and their partner which may result in relationship changes. Spouses who are actively involved in their partner's treatment plan often report that they receive more emotional support than spouses who were not involved. Partners can report feelings of loneliness because healthcare professionals focus on the individual and their immediate treatment. After the postoperative period and rehabilitation, life begins to become normalised and the partners become stronger. Pazar et al (2015) report that nearly all of their respondents (96%) had no problem showing their body to their spouse. Reassuringly most considered that their spouse accepted their change in body image.

Family support

As early as the 1950s Dyk and Sutherland (1956) were interested in the psychological impact of colostomy formation. They considered that the family had an important part to play as they may help the individual to restore their social function. A diagnosis that requires formation of a stoma is an outcome that will affect the everyday lives of many family members of the individual.

Family members are among the most important resource for individuals coping with a stoma. Families have similar information needs to the individual undergoing surgery and they want this information to come from the healthcare professionals who are working with the individual.

Multicultural care

The delivery of healthcare does not happen in a vacuum. Health is very much part of a person's life that will involve upbringing, culture and faith. One of today's challenges in stoma care is to bring to a multicultural society a high quality of care that will meet the needs of the patient. To understand cultural awareness the nurse must remember that the uniqueness of groups has limitations as variation within any community is likely to be broad.

Disease incidence resulting in stoma formation appears to be lower in Black and Minority Ethnic (BME) populations in first generation émigrés. However, second and third generations who have been integrated into British society are showing more prevalence of diseases that may give rise to stoma formation such as ulcerative colitis (Williams 2006).

Muslim patients

Islam is a monotheistic faith embracing Allah as the one God, who is creator of the universe and the sacred book of Islam is the Qur'an (Koran). In examining religious worship in Muslims and their belief structure it was seen that a stoma could significantly interfere with religious rituals and activities. Muslims follow the five pillars of Islam; one that can be affected by having a stoma is Salah or ritual praying five times a day. To take part in prayers a

Muslim must ensure that their clothes, body and place of prayer are clean, achieved by ablution (Al-Wadhu) before prayer, following sexual relations, urination and defecation. Having a stoma can negatively affect Muslims' quality of life and their willingness to continue participation in religious rituals and activities.

The passing of uncontrolled faeces or flatus negates the ablution. In patients with a stoma, social activity can be significantly impaired because some people stop praying at the mosque or even praying alone after surgery. During worship a series of movements are undertaken including standing, kneeling, bowing and touching the ground with the forehead when kneeling. This has great importance when siting a person for a stoma before their operation. In discussing with Muslim patients where they would like the stoma to be sited, below or above the umbilical area, many will say above the umbilical area as it will be considered 'clean' (Black 2000). Having a stoma raised for a life threatening disease or trauma should not cause any religious or cultural problems (Henley and Schott 1999). A determination of the legal ruling by the Board of the Mission Council in Indonesia was sought for patients who had a stoma.

Many Muslims will eat a strict vegetarian diet when they are away from home, although they will eat Halal meat, and alcohol is forbidden. Fasting is required for 28 days during Ramadan, with no food, fluid or medication being allowed to be consumed between the hours of sunrise and sunset. For patients with an ileostomy this can be very difficult as the patient may become dehydrated. Furthermore, eating a large meal late in the evening can disrupt stoma output. During the summer months the fasting period is much longer than during the winter months due to the longer hours of daylight. Some Muslim patients may decline surgery during Ramadan preferring to wait.

Sikh patients

Sikhism is very much a community focused religion with charity and community service encouraged. There are approximately twenty million followers throughout the world. Sikhs should not have their hair cut or bodily hair removed unless it is really necessary and then only a minimum should be removed. The ceremonial dagger is often a symbolic one but this may cause concern and a security problem in hospital if the understanding of the religion is limited. White shorts are worn by men and are kept on at all times. If they need to be changed one leg should always be kept in the shorts and each leg changed around individually and not removed in total. Sikh women may wish to keep their head covered with a shawl or scarf even when in hospital. Women prefer to be examined by a female and many Sikh husbands will insist on this. Medication such as loperamide capsules or antibiotic capsules can be difficult as they are made from animal gelatine and Sikhs require vegetarian gelatine.

Hindu patients

There are approximately 700 million Hindus in India and twenty million elsewhere in the world. It is a diverse religion and is considered more a way of life than a religion. Many people pray three times a day also before meals and sleep. Often they sit on the floor or may sit on the hospital bed crossed leg to pray. Some Hindus meditate, some practice yoga and many combine these. Modesty is a religious requirement and the head is regarded as sacred and not touched by others without permission. Food restrictions vary within Hinduism. Running water must be used for cleansing and using the toilet and keeping clean can cause great anxiety for Hindu patients in hospital. Incontinence and suppurating wounds can also cause great distress. Hindus are not allowed to take medication that is in gelatine as it is generally from an animal (cow) and is therefore prohibited. Vegan capsule medication will be needed.

References

Ang SG, Chen HC, Siah RJ, He HG, Klainin-Yobas P (2013) Stressors relating to patient psychological health following stoma surgery: an integrated literature review. Oncology Nursing Forum. 40(6): 587–594.

Annon JS (1976) The PLISSIT model: a proposed conceptual scheme for the behavioural treatment of sexual problems. Journal of Sex Education and Therapy. 2(1): 1–15.

Association of Stoma Care Nurses UK (2015) Stoma care nursing standards and audit tool. ASCN UK. London.

Berry J, Black P, Smith R, Stuchfield B (2007) Assessing the value of silicone and hydrocolloid products in stoma care. British Journal of Nursing. 16(13): 778–88

Black P (2013) The role of accessory products in patients with a stoma. British Journal of Nursing. 22(5): S24.

Black P (2000) Holistic Stoma Care. Ballière Tindall, London.

Borwell B (2009) Rehabilitation and stoma care: addressing the psychological needs. British Journal of Nursing. 18(4): S20–S25.

Cottam J and Richards K (2006) National audit of stoma complications within 3 weeks of surgery. Gastrointestinal Nursing. 4(8): 34–39.

Cowin C and Redmond C (2012) Living with a parastomal hernia. Gastrointestinal Nursing. 10(1): 16–24.

David GG, Slavin JP, Willmott S, Corless DJ, Khan AU et al (2010) Loop ileostomy following anterior resection: is it really temporary? Colorectal Disease. 12(5): 428–432.

Dyk RB and Sutherland AM (1956) Adaptation of the spouse and other family members to the colostomy patient. Cancer. 9(1):123–38.

Furukawa C, Sasaki Y, Matsui K, Morioka I (2013) Health-related quality of life and its relevant factors in Japanese patients with a urostomy. Journal of Wound Ostomy and Continence Nursing. 40(2): 165–170.

Galloway SC and Graydon JE (1996) Uncertainty, symptom distress, and information needs after surgery for cancer of the colon. Cancer Nursing. 19(2): 112–117.

Gianotten WL, Bender JL, Post MW and Höing M (2006) Training in sexology for medical and paramedical professionals: a model for rehabilitation setting. Sexual and Relationship Therapy. 3(21): 303–317.

Goodhart F, Atkins L (2011) The cancer survivor's companion: practical ways to cope with your feelings after cancer. London: Piatkus.

Henley A and Schott J (1999) Culture, religion and patient care in a multi-ethnic society. Age Concern. London.

Jackson C and Barnwall A (2014) Reversal of ileostomy following elective anterior resection for rectal cancer: a review of current practice. Gastrointestinal Nursing. 12(1): 23–30.

Kiliç E, Taycan O, Belli AK, Ozmen M (2007) The effect of permanent ostomy on body image, self-esteem, marital adjustment, and sexual functioning. Turk Psikiyatri Derg. 18(4): 302–10.

Kristensen SA, Laustsen S, Kiesbye B and Jensen BT (2013) The urostomy education scale: a reliable and valid tool to evaluate urostomy self-care skills among cystectomy patients. Journal of Wound Ostomy and Continence Nursing. 40(6): 611–617.

Krouse RS, Herrinton LJ, Grant M et al (2009) Health-related quality of life among long-term rectal cancer survivors with an ostomy: manifestations by sex. Journal of Clinical Oncology. 27(28): 4664–70.

Liu NW, Hackney JT, Gelhaus PT, Monn MF, Masterson TA et al (2014) Incidence and risk factors of parastomal hernia in patients undergoing radical cystectomy and ileal conduit diversion. The Journal of Urology. 191: 1313–1318.

Lyon CC and Smith A (2009) Abdominal stomas and their skin disorders. Second edition. Informa Healthcare. Florida, USA.

McKenzie F, White CA, Kendall S, Finlayson A, Urquhart M et al (2006) Psychological impact of colostomy pouch change and disposal. British Journal of Nursing. 15(6): 308–316.

McPhail J, Nichols T and Menier M (2014) A convex urostomy pouch with adhesive border: a patient survey. British Journal of Nursing. 23 (22): 1182–1186.

Notter J and Bernard P (2006) Preparing for loop ileostomy surgery: women's accounts from a qualitative study. International Journal of Nursing Studies. 43:147–159.

Ozturk O, Murat Yalcin B, Unal M, Yildirim K, Ozlem N (2015) Sexual dysfunction among patients having undergone colostomy and its relationship with self-esteem. Journal of Family Medicine & Community Health. 2(1):1028.

Persson E, Gustavsson B, Hellström AL, Lappas G and Hultén L (2005) Ostomy patients' perceptions of quality of care. Journal of Advanced Nursing. 49(1): 51–58.

Porrett T and McGrath A (2005) Stoma care. Blackwell Publishing. Oxford.

Pringle W and Swan E (2001) Continuing care after discharge from hospital for stoma patients. British Journal of Nursing. 10(19): 1275–1288.

Ramirez M, McMullen C, Grant M, Altschuler A, Hornbrook MC et al (2009) Figuring out sex in reconfigured body: experiences of female colorectal cancer survivors with ostomies. Women Health. 49(8): 608–624.

Ratcliff CR, Scarano KA and Donovan AM (2005) Descriptive study of peristomal complications. Journal of Wound, Ostomy and Continence Nursing. 32(1): 33–37.

Thompson MJ and Trainor B (2007) Prevention of parastomal hernia: a comparison of results 3 years on. Gastrointestinal Nursing. 5(3): 22–28.

Thompson MJ and Trainor B (2005) Incidence of parastomal hernia before and after a prevention programme. Gastrointestinal Nursing. 3(20): 23–27.

Wade (1989) A Stoma is for Life. Scutari Press. London.

Williams J (2006) Sexual health: case study of a patient who has undergone stoma formation. British Journal of Nursing. 15(14): 760–763.